This I Believe

A hundred years from now it
will not matter where I lived,
where *I worked* or where I've been,
but the world may be different
because I was important in
contributing to a child's education.
Teeth that will last a lifetime
Begin with early prevention.

– anonymous author with additions by Lori Gagliardi

Dedication

This edition is dedicated with a heart full of love and thankfulness to
My husband,
who has unlimited energy, love,
commitment and support for me,

and

My two sons,
may your lives always be filled
with love, laughter, happiness and an
appreciation for education

and

Those special people that continue to "make a difference" in the lives of others by encouraging them to save their smiles.

Dental Health Education

Lesson Planning and Implementation

Second Edition

Lori Gagliardi
CDA, RDA, RDH, M.Ed.

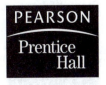

PEARSON

Prentice
Hall

Upper Saddle River, New Jersey 07458

Library of Congress Cataloging-in-Publication Data
Gagliardi, Lori.
    Dental health education: lesson planning and implementation /
Lori
  Gagliardi. — 2nd ed.
      p. ; cm.
    Includes bibliographical references.
    ISBN-13: 978-0-13-171738-1 (pbk.)
    ISBN-10: 0-13-171738-3
    1. Dental health education.   I. Title. [DNLM: 1. Health Education, Dental. 2. Teaching—methods.

  WU 113 G135d 2007]
  RK60.8.G34 2007
  617.6′01071—dc22   2006007758

Notice: The author and the publisher of this book have taken care to make certain that the equipment and schedules of treatment are correct and compatible with the standards generally accepted at the time of publication. Nevertheless, as new information becomes available, changes in treatment and in the use of equipment and procedures become necessary. The reader is advised to consult carefully the instruction and information material included in each piece of equipment or device before administration. Students are warned that the use of any techniques must be authorized by their medical advisor, where appropriate, in accordance with local laws and regulations. The publisher disclaims any liability, loss, injury, or damage incurred as a consequence, directly or indirectly, of the use and application of any of the contents of this book.

Publisher: Julie Levin Alexander
Executive Editor: Mark Cohen
Associate Editor: Melissa Kerian
Editorial Assistant: Nicole Ragonese
Managing Production Editor: Patrick Walsh
Production Liaison: Christina Zingone
Production Management/Composition: Chitra Ganesan/GGS Book Services
Manufacturing Manager: Ilene Sanford
Manufacturing Buyer: Pat Brown
Senior Design Coordinator: Maria Guglielmo
Cover Designer: Amy Rosen
Director of Marketing: Karen Allman
Senior Marketing Manager: Harper Coles
Printer/Binder: Bind-Rite Graphics
Cover Printer: Phoenix Color Corporation
Cover Credit: Randy Faris/Corbis-NY

Pearson Education LTD.
Pearson Education Australia PTY, Limited
Pearson Education Singapore, Pte. Ltd
Pearson Education North Asia Ltd
Pearson Education Canada, Ltd.
Pearson Educación de Mexico, S.A. de C.V.
Pearson Education–Japan
Pearson Education Malaysia, Pte. Ltd
Pearson Education, Inc., Upper Saddle River, New Jersey

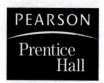

10 9 8 7 6 5 4 3 2
ISBN 0-13-171738-3

Contents

Preface

Dental disease is the most widespread public health problem among the school-age population in the United States today. In some states, 95 percent of children have dental disease in the form of dental caries and gingivitis. Dental disease in a child can and does result in significant lifetime and dental disability, dental pain, bleeding gums, missing teeth, time lost from school and work, and the need for dentures. Poor nutrition can also be a contributing factor.

Dental disease in children and the resultant abnormalities in adults can be prevented by education and treatment programs, beginning at an early age. Community dental disease prevention programs can be established for schoolchildren in kindergarten through sixth grade and in classes for children with special needs by local dental health professionals, volunteers, and students in the health care professions. Educational programs should focus on the development of personal practices by students that promote dental health and self awareness. Topics to be emphasized would include causes and prevention of dental diseases, nutrition, dental health and safety, and the need for regular visits to the dental office. The goals of a dental disease prevention program in the classroom are to:

- Instill self-awareness and responsibilities in dental health.
- Encourage decision making about dental health issues.
- Enable students to develop appropriate skills to prevent dental disease.
- Instill positive values and attitudes about dental health to ensure lifelong learning.

A comprehensive dental health program in the classroom is based on the concept of the "whole child," in which dental health is viewed as an integral part of total body health. Through this approach, it is hoped that learning about dental health will be integrated as part of students' school-based education rather than being merely a fragmented portion of classroom instruction.

To meet the goals described above, classroom lessons presented in an organized manner have proven to be the most effective approach. Learning good habits requires a change in behavior. Constant practice, repetition, and reinforcement are necessary. The information given must be the same for every child, otherwise the result will be merely confusion; no learning will take place. Changing students' oral hygiene habits, values, and attitudes toward dental health is the best—as well as the most cost-effective—way to solve dental health problems among the school-age population.

The second edition of *Dental Health Education* builds upon the first edition by presenting the most current information on topics such as nutrition and fluoride, as well as additional lesson plans, a section on adults, samples of teacher critiques, and new teaching ideas. There are now four sections:

Section One addresses the roles of the dental health educator and issues you should be aware of before planning and implementing your presentations. Before you begin, keep in mind that it is the responsibility of the dental health educator to be aware of the various factors that influence learning and behavioral change: The learning level of the targeted students, classroom environment, cultural factors, language barriers, amount of time available, and so forth. These are some of the factors you will need to address before entering the classroom. The more knowledgeable you are about the specific group to whom you are presenting, the better able you will be to deliver an effective presentation.

Section Two emphasizes and approaches for integrating dental health into the regular academic curriculum, and the development of visual aids to assist you in your presentations. This section provides suggestions to help you keep dental health education alive in the classroom throughout the year and to prevent fragmented learning. The goal is to ensure that dental health is not only addressed when dental health educators are present.

The lesson plans are organized using Hunter's (1977) five-step lesson plan, modified to include a preparation segment at the beginning and a time frame to keep you on track. The following format is used throughout this text:

- Preparation (things to do before beginning the lesson)
- Anticipatory planning (introduction of the lesson and materials needed)
- General objectives (what students will gain from the lesson)
- Instruction/information (the bulk of the lesson that is new and exciting for students)
- Guided practice activities (to reinforce the information taught)
- Closure (restatement of the objectives to test knowledge)

Also included in Section Two is information on targeting a special needs classroom.

Section Three presents the actual content of the dental health education program. In this text, dental health topics are broken up into lesson plans covering 11 essential areas of dental health education:

- The importance of plaque control
- Brushing for good oral health
- Flossing for good oral health
- The use of fluoride
- Nutrition and healthy teeth
- Dental sealants
- Dental safety and oral injury prevention
- Anti-tobacco lessons
- The dental office visit
- Last visit wrap up and review
- Children with special needs.

Section Four is a new section titled Creating a Community Outreach Program. It includes coverage of adult learners, low-literacy learners, the adult lesson plan, and oral health of older Americans.

Presentation of each lesson should take approximately 30 Minutes. All of the information for presenting a lesson, suggested activities, and individual lesson plan outline are included for each topic. It will be up to the reader to determine the students' current learning level, and what goals and objectives are obtainable. Therefore, information from the objectives (at the corresponding grade level) may be added to or deleted as needed. Lesson plans and information (e.g., plaque control and brushing) may also be combined into one lesson. However, I would caution against combining more than two topics in any one lesson plan.

This section is followed by an appendix of additional resources and a glossary. The appendix provides additional resources: The California Dental Association's fact sheets on dental care, tooth-talking vocabulary words, and a listing of additional dental health educational resources.

When I polled users of the first edition for recommended changes, additions, and modifications the first response was to leave it like it is. However, as time went on, many educators suggested more examples of lesson plans, a section for the special population of seniors, a teacher critique and any new information or ideas for teaching dental health education. All of these suggestions have been incorporated into the second edition. As my research continued, I also found opportunities to enhance the book's content on nutrition and fluoride. The result of this revision is an up-to-date resource that I hope will prove to be a valuable tool for you and the people you serve.

My thanks and gratitude for those of you that continue to make a difference in the lives of others by encouraging them to save their smiles, as teeth can last forever.

About the Author

Lori has been involved in dentistry since 1978. She began her career in dentistry graduating from the Pasadena City College Dental Assisting Program in 1979 and working at the USC School of Dentistry until 1988. In 1990 she completed her BS in Dental Hygiene at the USC School of Dentistry. In 1995 she completed her Masters Degree in Education and is currently a Doctorate Candidate in Organizational Leadership and Education at the University of La Verne (Ed.D) in California.

Her background and experience in education includes her current position as the program director for the Dental Assisting Program at Pasadena City College, Pasadena, California. In addition to program director duties, she teaches dental assistance and dental hygiene courses. She has had experience in private practice, public health, sealant clinics, education and consulting in addition to serving on many advisory boards for dental assisting, dental hygiene and dental health initiatives. She has written journal articles in radiology and dental materials.

Since 1990 she continues to play an active role in the local, state, and national dental hygiene organizations. She is a past president for both state (CDHA) and the local dental hygiene associations and has served in many appointed and elected positions as well. When she has time available, she enjoys traveling, reading, and spending time with family and friends.

Acknowledgments

I would like to acknowledge that much of this information is carried over from the 1st edition and a special thank you to those contributing again. In addition to the special friends and contributors to the 1st edition the following individuals have contributed and were a tremendous help in providing me with information and examples for this edition.

Marie Nieto-Grant, BS, MA, Project Manger Dental Health, CA Childrens' Dental Disease Prevention Program, Los Angeles County Office of Education
M. Diane Melrose, RDH, BS, USC School of Dentistry
Catherine Heinlein, RD, MS, CDE
Mark Bergman, FlossBrite, Bergman Oral Care, Chino, CA
Dave McCombs, FlossBrite, Bergman Oral Care, Chino, CA
Kristy Menage Bernie, RDH, BS, Educational Designs, Owner
Michelle Hurlbutt, RDH, BS
Charlotte Burruso, RDHAP, Visiting Dental Hygiene Services
Debra Doxey, RDH, MPH, Pasadena City College, Dental Hygiene Program
Thomas Neiderer, RDH, MPH, Pasadena City College, Dental Hygiene Program
Jeanne Porush, RDH, MFA, Pasadena City College, Dental Hygiene Program
Pasadena City College Dental Hygiene Students, Pasadena, CA
Patricia Stewart, RDH, ED, Cerritos College Dental Hygiene Program
Cerritos College Dental Hygiene Students, Cerritos CA
Joyce Flieger, Arizona Department of Health Services

Finally, thanks to Mark Cohen, Christina Zingone of Pearson, Chitra Ganesan and the staff at GGS Book Services for their hard work and dedication to this edition of Dental Health Edition, Lesson Planning and Implementation.

Reviewers

Lori Strunck, RDH, BS
Dental Assisting Education
Berdan Institute
Totowa, New Jersey

Thomas P. Neiderer, RHD, MPH
Assistant Professor, Dental Hygiene
Pasadena City College
Pasadena, California

Debby Kurtz-Weidinger, RDH, M.Ed.
Faculty, Dental Hygiene
Phoenix College
Phoenix, Arizona

Kim A. Norris, RDH, BA
Instructor, Dental Health
Carl Sandberg College
Galesburg, Illinois

Gayle McCombs, RDH, MS
Director and Associate Professor, Dental Hygiene
Old Dominion University
Norfolk, Virginia

Leah MacPherson, RDH, BS
Associate Professor, Dental Hygiene
Middlesex Community College
Lowell, Massachusetts

Before You Begin

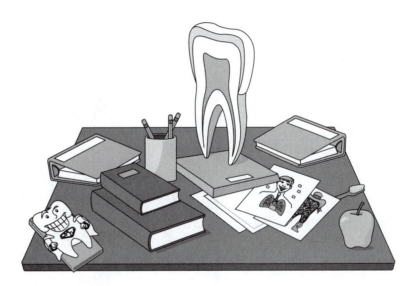

This section covers the roles of the dental hygienist or the dental health professional as the dental health educator in the community and discusses issues you should be aware of before planning and implementing your presentation. As emphasized in the introduction, Before You Begin, you should review factors that influence intrinsic behavior changes, multicultural issues, teaching methods, emotional and physical development of children in grades K–6, special needs, senior care, classroom presentation, community dental health programs, and classroom management. Remember, the more knowledge you have about the specific group to whom you will be presenting, the better able you will be to deliver an effective message.

CHAPTER 1

Community Dental Health Education

Many dental hygiene students picture themselves after graduation working for a general dentist or a periodontist as the preventive dental health specialist providing services for several patients each day. However, at some point in your career, you may wish to add a little variety to the daily office routine.

Dental hygienists were originally thought of and trained as oral health educators. Over the years, hygienists have been utilized in this capacity by working in settings such as schools, hospitals, nursing homes, general industry, public health facilities, and so on. Although in any of these settings hygienists may spend some time performing preventive services, the majority of their time probably is spent in education and administration.

It was common in the 1950s and 1960s to encounter dental hygienists who were employed part-time or full-time by local school districts. Often, a mobile "dental trailer" was set up at a school, where children received dental health instruction and were screened for dental decay. Local dentists then followed up with either free or low-cost dental care for the needy. As federal funding dwindled, these positions were eliminated for the most part in the western United States. The eastern states were more fortunate; local funding and support there have enabled many local dental health programs, coordinated by salaried dental hygienists, to continue their operations with additional dental hygiene preventive services.

Today, dental health is receiving a higher priority at the national level, and more state funding is being allocated for local dental health programs. Elementary schools have been targeted from the 1990s and into the future to meet the *Healthy People 2000, 2010* objective of decreasing dental disease among U.S. children.

Community involvement is an essential aspect of a professional career. Now is the time to become involved in the future by educating children in ways to prevent and eliminate dental disease. You can play a vital role as an educator in community dental health programs wherever you live.

Before becoming an active participant in a dental health program, you will need to become familiar with the issues that are discussed in the following pages.

WHAT IS A COMPREHENSIVE DENTAL HEALTH PROGRAM?

A comprehensive dental health program is based on the concept of teaching the "whole child," emphasizing dental health as an integral part of total body health. Through this approach, it is hoped that learning about dental health will not be merely a fragmented portion of instruction but instead will be integrated throughout a lifetime of learning

WHY ATTEMPT SUCH A COMPREHENSIVE, TIME-CONSUMING PROGRAM?

In the past few years, the dental community has expressed an increasing interest in school dental health. However, because of a lack of funding, most involvement has been on a volunteer basis. Typically, a dentist, dental hygienist, or dental health professional wishing to serve the community, volunteers to visit from one to many classrooms during the course of a school year. In such nonpaying programs, the participants' time commitment was often minimal, so classroom instruction was usually given as a "one-shot" presentation to as many children as possible. No matter how good the intentions of these volunteers, this type of instruction has been proven to be ineffective for several reasons:

- Constant practice, repetition, and reinforcement are necessary. Learning good oral hygiene habits requires a change in behavior. For instance, daily brushing and flossing have been shown to have a positive effect on dental health.
- The information given must be the same for every child. Otherwise, the result will be merely confusion; no learning will take place. Children often receive misinformation about dental health at home, so consistency at school is of the utmost importance.
- Any effective program needs to coordinate scheduling, supplies, evaluations, and so on. Volunteers generally do not have the time to take on these tasks.
- Follow-up referrals for emergency and preventive services are needed. Because of financial considerations, most dentists today are simply unable to render services to all needy families at a reduced cost. This service is usually provided by dental clinics—if parents have the necessary transportation and finances to utilize these services and recognize the importance of seeking needed dental care.

WHO IS INVOLVED IN A COMPREHENSIVE DENTAL HEALTH PROGRAM?

The following school personel will need to be involved in your program:

- Superintendent of schools
- Principal
- Health services coordinator
- School nurse
- Classroom teacher
- Local dental, dental hygiene, or dental health professional
- PTA/school support groups

The following community personel will need to be involved in your program:

- Community center administator
- Local society of dentists, dental hygienists, or dental health professional
- Volunteers
- Other health care providers affiliacted with the community center

Changing students' oral hygiene habits is the best way to solve the public health problem of dental disease among the school-age population. However, changing these habits involves factors that are intrinsic to behavioral change: knowledge, attitudes, values, and motivation. Table 1–1 can help you to identify your own intrinsic behaviors. Once you have established your own intrinsic behaviors, use this table to assess how you will create behavioral changes within the population for whom you will be providing dental health education.

Table 1–1   Factors That Influence Intrinsic Behaviors

Knowledge	Statistics show that only about 40% of the population visit the dentist in any one year, many of those only for relief of pain. It would seem that lack of knowledge is the most logical reason for the majority of the population not seeking preventive dental care. However, this is not the case. Today, as we teach dental health concepts to either individual patients or groups, many other factors must be taken into consideration. Some variables include social, cultural, economic, and demographic attributes. A false assumption is that increasing a person's dental health knolwledge will help change dental behavior.
Attitudes	This refers to the reactions of an individual to the learning he or she acquires. Attitudes develop slowly through a continuum of low-level experiences or suddenly, from one intense experience. Learned behavior stems from attitudes.
Values	Values usually refer to what a person feels is right or should be done. Every individual establishes a priority of value based on past experiences, which will influence his or her behavior. Even young children may demonstrate attitudes and values developed by modeling parents and teachers. Further, behavior change may take a lot longer for one child than another. Health educators also have attitides and values that influence their behavior and the aspects of helath instruction they emphasize. An educator must consider his or her own points of view relative to helath and education. What do you value in relation to dental helath and dental health education?
Motivation	The process of motivation involves the following steps: • A specific need • Action/behavior by the individual • A goal to be achieved • Some form of satisfaction

Multicultural Issues in Dental Health

Educators in today's classrooms are presented with a tremendously diverse student population. According to the Los Angeles County Office of Education, 90 languages are spoken in just that one area of the state. Each of these languages represents cultural as well as language barriers when it comes to communicating a dental health lesson in the classroom. Dental health educators must be sensitive to the needs of the ever-growing diversity of cultural backgrounds present in the classroom.

Communication and cultural diversity are closely interwoven. Communication, as defined by *Merriam–Webster's Collegiate Dictionary* (1993), refers to "a process by which information is exchanged between individuals through a common system of symbols, signs, or behavior." Culture is defined as "the customary beliefs, social norms, and material traits of a racial, religious, or social group." For many students, the information on dental health that is presented in the classroom may be very different from the culturally influenced teaching they have received within their family or community.

It can be said that most cultures have five major components:

1. A pattern of communication
2. A basic diet
3. A common style of dress
4. Common socialization patterns
5. A common set of values and beliefs

Cultural diversity influences how individuals express themselves, both verbally and nonverbally. Cultural patterns are embedded beginning at birth in childrearing practices. The communication practices of individual cultures affect the expression of ideas, feelings, and decision making. Variations in communication practices may be widespread (e.g., common to an entire cultural group), or limited to the use of particular words or gestures with specific meanings for a small group (e.g., the family). In addition, within a given culture is a set of values and beliefs that guide members' social communication.

What is accepted in one culture may be entirely inappropriate in another. For instance, Anglo-Americans may be more likely to conceal feelings than persons from other cultural groups, and the United States, in general, is considered a low-touch culture. In comparison, a member of a Middle-Eastern or Mediterranean culture may be open and loud with expressions, and rely on touch as an important part of communication. Similarly, the dominant American cultural values emphasize competition and individual achievement whereas many other cultures emphasize cooperation and group achievement.

The following example illustrates how this information can be applied to dental health education. Suppose you wanted to test the knowledge of a group of students. You might choose to question the students individually. However, suppose that their cultural background is one that emphasizes group achievement. In this instance, the classroom response to the dental health lesson would probably be very low. The educator must always remember that a dental health program that has been presented successfully to one class or group may have to be modified to fit another group. Cultural characteristics, language barriers, and a preference for cooperative rather than individual learning will all influence the educator's task. Thus, the educator should attempt to adapt the content and teaching methods of the lesson to meet the needs of the particular group of students.

Finally, remember that although all of us are influenced by our cultures, we remain individuals. It is difficult to accurately describe the characteristics of any cultural group, particularly as each new generation has an influence on its culture. When the dental health educator is sensitive to all cultures that may be represented in the classroom, he or she will be most effective in presenting information that can be absorbed by all students.

Additional information on putting together a complete dental public health program can be found at the American Dental Hygienists' Association (ADHA) website at www.adha.org, Public Health section: "ADHA Handbook for Dental Public Health Activities."

Integrating Dental Health Education into the Classroom

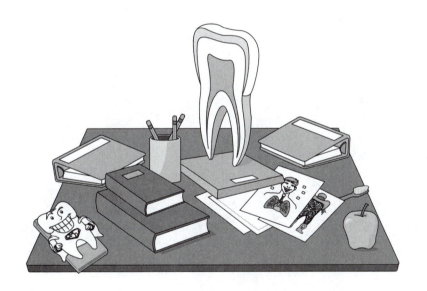

CHAPTER 2

Teaching Methods

Many different strategies can be used in teaching, among them: lecture, demonstration, discussion, inquiry, games, and activities. Not all can be handled effectively by everyone. Practice at least three of the methods that follow to determine which ones best fit your style and personality. As always, be sure the information presented is appropriate to the cognitive and physical level of the participants as outlined in Table 2–1.

LECTURE

The most traditional teaching method, lecture, is probably the easiest for the dental health educator who needs to simply develop material, memorize it, and deliver it verbatim to the class. Unfortunately, this method does not always ensure the level of learning desired. This failure to meet educational goals may stem from:

- A monotone style of presentation that fails to hold listeners' attention.
- A learning experience that is passive rather than active.
- A format that does not lend itself to questions, feedback, or discussion.

Among educators today, there is a tendency to depart from the traditional lecture format by using an entirely different approach or combining this method with one or two others.

DEMONSTRATION

As a teaching method, demonstration can be an effective tool, especially if the students' interest has been previously stimulated. Most often this method is combined with lecture, which has the advantage of involving two senses (hearing and seeing) instead of just one. Problems associated with demonstration include:

- Materials that are too cumbersome to carry with you
- For large groups, the need for special facilities so that everyone can see the demonstration
- Inability for one person to do the demonstration alone

When teaching dental health, demonstration becomes a key element in each presentation. You will want to perfect this method before focusing on others. Audiovisual (AV) aids fit into this category. Keep in mind as technology advances (PowerPoint, DVD, etc.), the participants' level of technology may or may not have advanced to the same level. Equipment may be limited at some sites, so be prepared to present your information with a variety of visuals to use in case what you were planning does not work.; i.e., you have everything on PowerPoint but no projector is available. Call ahead when possible and confirm type of AV available on site, outlet space, etc.

DISCUSSION

Control of the class is a major determinant of success or failure when employing discussion. This teaching method is usually most effective in small groups. An introductory lecture, demonstration, research assignment, or group sharing of

Table 2–1 Emotional and Physical Development of Children

Age/Grade	Emotional Characteristics	Physical Characteristics
5/Kindergarten	Very direct	Skips, hops
	Very interested in health problems and "why"	Laces shoes
	Enjoys talking	Fastens buttons
	Personal	Likes to copy
	Realistic	Holds a toothbrush
	Accepts help	Swishes without swallowing
	Basically kind	
6/First grade	Explores everything	Awkward in find motor tasks
	Easily distracted	Musch oral activity: blows, bites lips, chews pencils
	Changes activity easily	Takes things apart
	Wants to succeed	Ties shoes
	Wants to obey rules	Copies more accurately
	Demanding and stubborn	
7/Second grade	Wants to be perfect	Enjoys pencils, drawing, writing
	Hoards time and attention	Balances better
	Sensitive feelings	Personal care is better: dresses easily, brushes hair and teeth
	Less distracted	
	Poor loser	
8/Third grade	Curious	Very active
	Listens and watches	Facter and smoother in finer motor activities
	More conscious of relationships	More graceful
	Curious about body, what cures disease, nature, what cures	Can ride a bike
	More dramatic	More social
	Likes clubs, rules	Manipulative skills improve
	Interests are short-lived	
	Argues	
	Needs help in care of possessions	
	Likes riddles	
9/Fourth grade	Self-motivated	Difficult to calm after an activity
	Does not enjoy routine tasks	More energy
	Interested in perfecting skills	
	Better able to perform self-appraisal	
	Can accept criticism and fairness	
	Reasonable	
	Responsible	
	Awed by self, own ideas, power and body	
10/Fifth grade	Has heroes, loyalties, interest in social justice	Enjoys team sports
	Likes secret clubs	Interested in exercising
	Interested in body and how it works	Wants big muscles
	Little concern about personal grooming and helath	
11/Sixth grade	Self-conscious about body and how it appears to others	Exercise is important
	Interest in body differences	
	Focus on personal health, grooming, and being in style	

dental experiences may be necessary to stimulate students' interest and prepare them for this activity. Be aware of using openended questions; when presenting to adults, you may get no responses or too many responses. Ask more specific "inquiry questions" like "How many of you saw a dentist or dental hygienist within the last six months?" to stimulate discussion.

INQUIRY

Inquiry—the technique of asking questions to stimulate learning—is probably the most effective teaching method. However, it requires a considerable amount of skill on the part of the educator. With this teaching method, the class is expected to achieve the highest level of learning through self-discovery and reflection. A major concept is that the learner is exposed to a certain degree of frustration, which stimulates the thinking process more than rote memorization.

Little information or direction is given initially. The teacher asks questions to help the learner solve his or her own problems. For example, a dental health educator who wishes to teach an elementary school class about what teeth are used for, might ask a series of questions, such as:

1. "Why do you suppose we have teeth?"—This first question will probably elicit some correct answers, but usually not all possibilities.
2. "Can you think of any other reasons we have teeth?"—At this point, the educator must allow ample time for the students to think through the question and produce additional answers.

If the educator had begun by saying, "We have teeth for several reasons. Teeth help us to chew our food, smile, talk, and so on," the children would be given some points to memorize. More than likely, they would be unable to remember all the answers a short time later. By using the inquiry method, however, the children are compelled to think about how they use their own teeth and then come up with the answers. Children who learn in this way are much more likely to remember the lesson. This technique will work with adults as well, just be mindful of the openended questions that may need to be more specific to narrow the response rate.

GAMES AND ACTIVITIES

If handled properly, games and activities can be incorporated into any of the previously mentioned teaching methods. To be successful, however, they must be well planned and organized with an objective in mind. This method is one of the best ways to stimulate interest and participation in the elementary school classroom.

Classroom Presentation

There are several aspects of classroom presentation that you will need to address before becoming an effective educator. These aspects may come naturally to you, or some or all aspects may be intermittently or continually frustrating. However, your efforts to master these aspects will improve your presentations.

INITIAL FEAR OF SPEAKING IN FRONT OF AN AUDIENCE

It is perfectly normal to be nervous or, in some cases, terrified when facing an audience. The best way to control this anxiety is to be well prepared for your presentation. Here are a few tips:

- Do not rely on reading notes.
- Do not rely on your partner to take over.
- Do prepare in front of an audience—this will help you feel comfortable and may also provide you with feedback on your speaking voice, level of enthusiasm, and body language.
- Do speak up! If you speak with assurance, the quiver in your voice will shortly disappear.
- Do practice! Out loud not just in your head. Work on your pitch, tone, volume, and timing.
- Do anticipate problems. Nothing is more unnerving than to plan to introduce a film only to find that the projector is broken or unavailable. Always rehearse an alternative plan and be sure additional equipment, if needed, is requested in advance.
- Do encourage questions from your audience. Their participation will allow you a moment to relax and let your heart stop pounding.
  - Show up early.
  - Talk to your students and do not read a script.
  - Know your audience: ask about previous dental knowledge of the group, what are their expectations, who are they, and why are they there.
  - Use humor that is appropriate, on target, and makes the point memorable.
  - Take care of yourself: eat something, drink water, avoid too much caffeine or stimulants. Take some deep breaths and visualize success.
  - Never apologize: be positive and comfortable with the quality of your materials.
  - Respect the audience: assume they are interested in the topic.
  - Listen carefully and answer questions thoughtfully.
  - Finish early: the audience will be appreciative.

    (Adapted from "Tips on Giving Effective Presentation," Washington State Department of Health Services.)

Initially, your presentations may be limited, for the most part, to a lecture that simply introduces facts. Once you begin to relax in front of the classroom, however, you can begin to think about other aspects of your presentation, such as audiovisual aids and interactive components.

QUALITY OF AUDIOVISUAL AIDS, DEMONSTRATION, AND/OR PARTICIPATION TECHNIQUES

When developing audiovisual aids or other interactive strategies for your presentation, keep the following points in mind:

- Do make sure everyone can see the demonstration, poster, or other display. Hold it up long enough for the participants to read or interpret the message.

- Walk around the classroom if necessary so that everyone can see.
- If you pass out materials, make sure everyone has a chance to see, hold, or feel the item before you move on to the next step.
- Try to establish eye contact with everyone in the room.
- Do not demonstrate toothbrushing, flossing, or other techniques on yourself *while* trying to give directions verbally.
- Make sure all participants begin a procedure together.
- Giving directions for a group procedure requires some thought. Be sure directions are clear and concise. You may need to repeat directions several times in the elementary school classroom.
- Be sure you have thoroughly demonstrated the expected behavior (e.g., holding the toothbrush properly and brushing in a sequence) before passing out supplies. This will ensure that the attention of the audience will be focused on you.
  - Use handouts (fact sheets are in the appendix section) to illustrate your points to give greater detail.
  - Overheads are used for small groups of 30 or less. Use only good quality images. Practice handling the overheads comfortably so you are not shuffling and dropping them. Number the overhead transparencies ahead of time in the order of the presentation sequence.
  - Slides are of higher quality and better than overheads for larger group presentations. Be careful not to put too much information on one slide. Photographic images can leave a memorable impression.
  - Short video clips can help to add interest. Do not forget about the special equipment that might be needed to run the video clips within your presentation.
  - Presentation software is a helpful tool. Using a data projector, your slides and overheads can be projected from a laptop. Be sure that the facilities have the appropriate equipment for your use. Be sure your disk, software, and equipment are compatible. Providing copies of the PowerPoint presentation is helpful and appreciated with the adult learners.
  - Charts and graphs can be very effective if well designed. Make them simple and easily grasped in a few seconds. Use them to show dramatic differences.

TEACHING CONCEPTS

Once your presentation is well under control, you will be able to scrutinize your message and the effectiveness of the communication. This would include the following:

- Be aware of classroom clues to noncommunication (such as talking, shuffling, and looking around the room).
- Summarize difficult concepts through demonstration, interpretive question and answer sessions, class discussions, and so on.
- Obtain the anticipated answer to your questions, rather than simply a "yes" or "no" response.
- Observe problems in brushing and flossing technique and correcting them immediately.
- Be an active listener and begin to answer questions spontaneously in more detail. At this point, some questions may allow you to explain a new concept without having to rely on a prepared script.
- Be aware of items in the classroom that can enhance your presentation. Often, teachers display projects related to dental health. These related materials provide an opportunity to: (1) compliment the class and/or

teacher, thus establishing rapport; (2) reinforce a concept already introduced; and (3) introduce a new concept by building on one already introduced.

MOTIVATION THROUGH FEELINGS

This aspect involves affective learning; helping students to express their feelings and attitudes, and perhaps reflect on or establish values related to dental health. Achieving this goal is difficult, particularly with younger elementary school children. Techniques to accomplish this would include:

- Role playing
- Structured values activities
- Learning games
- Small group interaction

Most of the activities throughout this book are geared toward motivating the class through experiences and feelings. Do not be afraid to be creative. Keep in mind, however, that the concepts you are teaching should remain consistent and appropriate for the grade level or the particular classroom.

AN EIGHT-STEP MODEL FOR PLANNING INSTRUCTION

After reviewing the preceding information, you should have a good idea of the specific techniques you want to use in your presentation to your targeted group. Now, you need to put your lesson plan together. You can begin by utilizing the eight-step planning model developed by Renner (1985). This model will also be used to incorporate more specific information that applies to Hunter's (1971) five-step lesson plan, which is presented in Section Two.

Determine Objectives: The easiest place to begin is to write down your goals and objectives for each presentation. Determine what you expect your students to be able to accomplish by the end of the lesson and how you would like them to consider responsibilites. Be specific with your objectives. Avoid generalities such as "the student will appreciate the value of good dental health." If your objectives are equally measurable, it will be easier to assess whether they have been met at the end of the presentation.

Assess Your Own Skills: By now you have an idea of what works for you—your teaching style. Plan your program around your personality, your attitudes, your knowledge, and your interests. Play on your individual strengths.

Determine the Learners' Skill: Seek out those who can give you insight (teachers) into the needs and abilities of your prospective students. Conference with the group contact person. Arrange a visit purely for observation. Talk to colleagues who have worked with this group or a similar group in the past. The better prepared you are, the easier it will be to plan and present the information that is of value to your audience. They will appreciate the fact that you did your homework and that you are able to relate to their specific level and needs.

Survey the System: The school, company, staff, institution, or other setting in which your program will take place often influences who attends, what is expected, and what is likely to happen. Discover any rules that may affect your presentation and any administrative constraints that may apply. Note the atmosphere of the facility (relaxed, stiff, formal, academic, happy, liberal, etc.).

Choose Appropriate Teaching/Learning Strategies: Certain strategies are more suitable for certain learning objectives. In general, a combination of demonstration, lecture, and plenty of practice yield desired results. Read the section on classroom presentation and determine what will work best for your group based on their needs, motivation, and abilities.

Incorporate Evaluation and Feedback: Build opportunities for frequent feedback into your presentation. Keep in mind that after you complete your self-evaluation or receive the evaluation from the contact person in a community outreach program, you can change or improve your presentation. Solicit feedback often throughout your presentations by asking such questions as:

- "Before I go on, does this make sense to you?"
- "Am I going too fast?"
- "Did I lose you?"
- "Are there any questions you want me to answer?"
- "You seem confused" (responding to nonverbal signs), "can I help?"

Try not to answer your own questions too often. Devise questions based on information and knowledge, making it difficult for students to answer with a simple "yes" or "no" response.

Provide for Restructuring: Allow for flexibility and change by keeping your lesson plans and ideas tentative and brief. Remember that your presentation is only a *proposed* outline. It may have to be changed as you become more familiar with your participants' needs and abilities.

ADDITIONAL PRESENTATION TECHNIQUES

Here are a few final tips that you can use to improve your presentations:

- Start your presentation on time and be prepared and have visual aids ready. When working with a partner, rehearse who will say what and when.
- Begin the lesson after the class has settled down and is ready to pay attention to you.
- Make sure the students can actually read before asking them to do so.
- Choose appropriate vocabulary. Younger children may be confused by words such as "tissues," "maintain," "promote," and so on.
- When passing items around the room for inspection, stop the lesson until all the items have been returned to you; otherwise you will lose your audience.
- Similarly, when resuming your lecture after an activity such as playing a game or coloring a handout, tell the children to put away these materials before continuing with the lesson.
- Use the blackboard whenever possible. Print or write using letters that match those the children are being taught, and write large enough so that all the students can read what you have written.
- Call on a variety or participants. There will always be one or two children who will raise their hands before you have even finished asking a question. Try waiting a bit longer, then say, "Let's give someone else [or another group/table] a chance."
- One of the most important elements in successful learning is making sure all the participants can hear what is being said. In most classes, a child's question will not be heard by any of the children sitting behind him or her. Always repeat the question beginning your answer. This also provides a chance to clarify or expand on the question.
- *Listen carefully to questions.* Oftentimes, questions give you a great opportunity to discuss or clarify an important concept. Remember, if one asks the question, many others may be thinking the same thing.

Classroom Management

Research has shown that students perform better academically when teachers are good classroom managers. Students in these situations learn and retain more than students of teachers who are not good classroom managers.

Teachers who are good classroom managers share the following traits. They:

- Are clear about their expectations and clearly present directions, objectives, and the purpose of the lesson.
- Present information in small steps.
- Allow students to practice.
- Monitor and provide feedback.
- Plan ahead by being prepared, establishing signals, taking charge, rewarding task-oriented behaviors, being positive, being specific, and providing immediate reinforcement.

In addition, these teachers:

- Stay calm.
- Deal with problems immediately.
- Have a secure routine.
- Teach at the correct level of difficulty.
- Are enthusiastic.
- Use humor.
- Speak at the right voice level.
- Use appealing visuals, which can be seen by everyone.
- Question and respond appropriately.
- Use a variety of teaching methods that appeal to three types of learners: auditory, visual, and kinesthetic.
- Use active participation techniques such as discussing with a partner, brainstorming, using signals (finger, thumb up, eye and hand motions), encouraging response in unison (everyone thumb up if you agree), including activities appropriate to children's motor development, getting one student to respond (agree or disagree), flashing answers to the group, and using flash cards.

By using these techniques, you can improve your own classroom management skills and enhance your ability to deliver effective dental health presentations to a variety of students.

KEY LEARNINGS

Once your presentation has been made, take time to reflect on how the presentation went.

Ask yourself the following questions:

- Was the presentation started on time?
- Was the information presented in an organized manner?
- Did the participants respond to the questions?
- Did the participants participate in the discussion?
- Was the activity/discussion relevant to the information presented?
- Do I need to provide the teacher/host with additional information?
- What did I learn from this experience?
- Has the teacher/host completed an evaluation on the presentation?
- Have I reviewed and compare the results with my own key learning?
- What changes should I make before the next presentation?

DENTAL HEALTH EDUCATION INSTRUCTOR EVALUATION

NAME OF PRESENTER(S) _____

DATE OF PRESENTATION _____ TOPIC _____

NAME AND LOCATION OF PRESENTATION SITE _____

GRADE LEVEL/AUDIENCE _____ TEACHER/COORDINATOR _____

GRADING CRITERIA   START TIME _____
9–10: EXCELLENT   FINISH TIME _____
7–8: VERY GOOD
5–6: GOOD
3–4: FAIR IMPROVEMENT NEEDED
2 or below: UNACCEPTABLE/REVISE INFORMATION IN THIS AREA

Criteria	Comments	Grade/Points
1. Presentation started and ended on time		10 8 6 4 2
2. Presentation was organized and presented in a sequential order		10 8 6 4 2
3. Information presented was appropriated for the audience/grade level		10 8 6 4 2
4. Visual aides were appropriate for the grade level and information presented		10 8 6 4 2
5. Objectives were stated		10 8 6 4 2
6. Activity was used to reinforce learning and check for knowledge		10 8 6 4 2
7. Time was given for participants to ask and answer questions		10 8 6 4 2
8. Presenters' demeanor/professionalism was appropriate		10 8 6 4 2
9. Presenters were knowledgeable in the subject area presented		10 8 6 4 2
10. Overall presentation		10 8 6 4 2
Total		

Possible points   100

Evaluator _____ Date _____
          Additional comments

LESSON PLAN

TOPIC _____

GRADE LEVEL _____ ROOM _____

SCHOOL _____ TEACHER _____

TIME REQUIRED _____

Preparation in classroom _____

_____

_____

_____

_____

Anticipatory planning _____

_____

_____

_____

_____

_____

_____

Review of previous objectives _____

_____

_____

_____

_____

Three specific objectives:

1. _____

_____

2. _____

_____

3. _____

_____

Lesson Plan continued

Information to Be Presented

Topics _____

_____

_____

_____

_____

_____

Guided-practice activities _____

_____

_____

_____

_____

_____

Closure _____

_____

_____

_____

_____

_____

Follow-up activity _____

_____

_____

_____

_____

_____

Reminder for the next visit: Date, time, topic, advanced preparation (if applicable)

_____

_____

_____

_____

_____

CHAPTER 3

Hints to Help Integrate the Dental Education Program

INTEGRATING DENTAL HEALTH EDUCATION INTO THE CLASSROOM

This section emphasizes different approaches to integrate dental health education into the regular academic curriculum and provides guidelines for developing visual aids that can assist you in your presentations. The goal is to develop informative activities and visuals that can be utilized by the classroom teacher and incorporated in classroom learning throughout the year. Dental health education is most effective when it is integrated into classroom activities and not fragmented or mentioned only when dental health educators are present.

Hints to Help Integrate the Dental Education Program Into the Academic Curriculum

Dental health concepts can be reinforced in several different areas of the elementary school curriculum. The following are suggested activities that can be utilized by teachers during creative writing, English, reading, social studies, math, and science/health portions of the curriculum.
—Arlene Globe, RDH

CREATIVE WRITING

- Have students write paragraphs on topics such as "My Life as a Tooth" or "My Life as a Loose Tooth."
- Have students create comic strips about teeth talking to each other about important dental health messages.
- Have the class write a commercial for a new and exciting dental product. Students may create artwork to go with the commercial, and a song or jingle to describe the product.
- Have students write a paragraph on their feelings about a trip to the dentist.
- Have students design and write about inventions that might help care for teeth.
- Have the class design a dialogue between two or three teeth. Encourage students to ask questions such as, What kind of tooth are you? Where do you live and who are your neighbors? Does it cost much to care for you?
- Have students write a scary story using characters such as the ghost-like Plaque and the evil Sweet Sugar. Illustrate the story.
- Valentine's Day, Christmas, Halloween, and Easter are times when children often overeat sweets. Ask children to write about a special holiday feast where something magical happened and good food choices were made.
- Divide students into groups. Have each group write a play about teeth. It can be fiction, nonfiction, or science fiction. Set aside one afternoon for the various performances. Supply healthy snacks as a treat.
- Research what's new in dentistry. Have students do a "News Bulletin" announcing the new discoveries.

ENGLISH

- Have students write a poem about teeth.
- Ask students to interview their parents about their dental experiences and then report back to the class.
- Create a dental spelling list (refer to the appendix listing of dental terms and the glossary at the end of this book). Have the students write different sentences using each word.
- Ask students to write a letter to their dentist describing how they take care of their teeth and asking if there are any other things they can do.
- Ask students to write about the dental health professionals in their dental office, including who they are and what they do.

READING

- Read one of the creative writing dental stories presented in Section 2. Have a discussion afterward. Have students draw or write about their favorite part of the story, or what they did or did not like about the story.
- Have students make up pictures and stories about teeth or another dental subject.

SOCIAL STUDIES

- Have students research the following topics: (1) how early settlers might have cared for their teeth, (2) the history of the toothbrush, (3) the history of dentistry, and (4) problems early settlers may have had with their teeth.
- Talk about changes in dental technology in the past 25-years. Then, have students write a report on these changes after interviewing their parents or a local dentist. Students should also be encouraged to use the school library for research.
- Have students make up their own laws about dental health and safety.
- Have students discuss how their eating patterns change when they are away from home (at camp, a relative's house, etc.). What kinds of things do they eat at camp? At their grandparents' house? When they are on vacation?
- Have students research the various ways that people from different periods of time or cultures have taken care of their teeth. The teacher may want to divide the class into groups and assign a different era or different country to each group.
- Have students design a map of a town with streets and public buildings. Have them place a real or fictional dental office on the map. Accompany the map with a short story about what goes on at a dental office or why we should go.

MATH

- Create word problems for all grade levels using dental words or objects.
- Write a few logic and reasoning stories that contain math problems relating to dental facts, nutrition, or other related areas.
- Have students make an "Acid Attack Chart" that lists every snack or meal eaten during the day. Add up the 20-minute periods after each snack or meal to get a total number indicating the amount of time acid is attacking the teeth. Make a graph of the information on the chart.

SCIENCE AND HEALTH*

- Make a poster of items that cause a lot of damage to the teeth. Try to design it so it sends a message without the use of words.
- Show students pictures of a healthy tooth and a decayed tooth. Ask students to create their own tooth out of clay or soap. Be sure to name all the parts of the tooth.
- Have students create a dental survey containing at least five questions relating to dental health. Tell them to ask at least 10 friends the questions, then bring the answers back to class and compare them. Have students write conclusions and recommendations from what they have learned.
- Make a hidden sugar display (see Chapter 8). Using common foods, ask students to add up the amount of sugar consumed in a day, a week, and a month.

* Prepared by the office of Dental Health, Maine Department of Human Services.

Science experiments are useful learning tools when working with students. Hands-on experiences have a lasting impact and illustrate concepts that are difficult to convey on paper. Four experiments that can be conducted in the classroom are described on the following pages.

Experiment 1: Spoiling Apple

This experiment uses the decaying process of apples to illustrate dental decay.

Supplies

- Two apples
- Bowl

Directions

First, place an apple with a tiny spot on it in a bowl. The tiny spot will spread through the whole apple, which is similar to the manner in which decay progresses through the tooth. Cutting the apple in half will illustrate this process for students.

Next, place an apple with a small bruise spot touching an apple that is not bruised. In time, the apple that had no spot will have a decay spot on it. This illustrates how decay on one tooth will spread to the tooth that it is touching.

Experiment 2: Egg and Vinegar

This experiment shows that acid weakens substances such as tooth enamel that contain calcium. It also shows that fluoride strengthens tooth enamel against acid, reinforcing the importance of brushing with fluoride toothpaste and receiving fluoride treatments regularly from the dental office.

Supplies

- Two hard boiled eggs
- A large empty pickle jar
- White vinegar
- A plastic food storage bag
- Fluoride gel (may obtained through your dentist or hygienist)

Directions

Take one egg and put it in the plastic bag containing the fluoride gel. Make sure that the fluoride completely covers the entire eggshell. Leave the egg in fluoride overnight. Then take both eggs and place them in a jar containing vinegar. Examine the eggs every few hours. As the acid from the vinegar attacks the egg, bubbles rise from it. Notice that one egg has more bubbles than the other. Leave the eggs overnight. Take both eggs out of the jar the next day and examine them. The shell of the egg that was placed in fluoride will be harder than that of the other egg.

Experiment 3: Effects of Acid on Teeth

This experiment illustrates how acid attacks tooth enamel, eventually leading to tooth decay.

Supplies

- Extracted tooth
- A small bottle
- White vinegar

Directions

Place an undecayed tooth in a bottle containing vinegar. The stronger the vinegar and the longer the time, the greater the effect on the tooth. As the acid demineralizes the tooth, the enamel loses its translucency, turns a chalky opaque white, and becomes soft. Eventually, the tooth will become so soft you will be able to pierce it with a needle. These changes in the tooth are similar to the process by which a tooth decays in the mouth.

Experiment 4: Tooth in Coke

This experiment illustrates how foods containing sugar cause teeth to decay.

Supplies

- Two jars
- A soft drink with high sugar content (e.g., Coca-Cola)
- A soft drink with a sugar substitute (e.g., Diet Coke, which has aspartame)
- Extracted teeth

Directions

Pour some of the soft drink into a jar. Add the undecayed tooth. Let the tooth remain in the jar for 4–6 months. This is a good experiment to do at the beginning of the school year. Students can note their observations throughout the year. Remove the tooth after 4–6-months. It should be soft and might crumble. Compare the difference from the tooth in the high sugar content jar with that in the sugar substitute jar. Discuss the results of soft drinks on teeth. High acidity is cariogenic despite the lack of sugar.

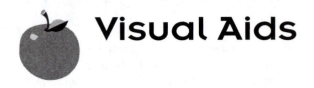

Visual Aids

CREATING AN APPROPRIATE VISUAL AIDS

Visual aids have several advantages in the classroom. They:

- Help the educator to present ideas exactly.
- Appeal to more than one sense.
- Broaden the learner's experience.
- Are suitable for all ages.
- Are effective when language barriers exist.

The purpose of the visual aid is to: (1) assist the educator in attaining the objective of the lesson, and (2) improve the learning situation and make it more meaningful. Among the various types of visual aids that can be used are:

- One dimensional
- Two dimensional
- Three dimensional
- Audiovisual
- Creative plays or games

Examples of each of these visual aids and ideas for using them in the classroom are presented below.

ONE-DIMENSIONAL VISUAL AIDS

One-dimensional visual aids include chalkboards or marker boards, charts, bulletin boards, flip charts, projected aids, and duplicated aids.

Chalkboard/Marker Board

This board can be planned and drawn before the start of the lesson, or if used spontaneously to explain a concept. It is available in most classrooms and can be especially effective when used with forethought.

Chart

A chart can be an effective aid, particularly when simple. When creating charts, focus on one idea and make it graphic. Use color to distinguish different points or areas of the chart.

Charts can be used to:

- Present data (e.g., percentages of children with tooth decay).
- Provide a schematic representation of an idea (e.g., the decay process).
- Diagram activities or information.
- Graph data.

Bulletin Board

A bulletin board is available in most classrooms and can be used to present a variety of ideas and materials. An effective bulletin-board display should project only one major idea. Use simple lettering and illustrations. The layout patterns can be symmetrical or diagonal.

Flip Chart

This is an inexpensive, permanent, and portable visual aid. Many types of preprinted flip charts are available, including flash cards, stories, and charts; or create your own using a large tablet—flip through pre-drawn pages or draw as needed.

Projected Aid

This category includes slides, single-concept films (usually between 2 and 4 minutes in length), PowerPoint™, and transparencies for use with an overhead projector. Slide or Power-Point™ programs have the advantages of being flexible, handy, and easily edited. Transparencies are easy to make. Be sure to check with the facilities ahead of time or bring your own projectors (LCD, laptop, slide projector, overhead unit).

Duplicated Aids

This category includes any handouts or visuals made with a photocopier or other duplicating system.

TWO-DIMENSIONAL VISUAL AIDS

Two-dimensional visual aids include flannel boards, Velcro boards, and self-stick lettering.

Felt Board

A felt board is a relatively inexpensive aid that is particularly effective for small children, enabling them to replay the story or lesson. The size of the board should reflect the number of students or attendees. Be sure that the board can be seen by all participants. Cover a large piece of light-weight wood or foam board with felt. Cut-out characters can have Velcro or sandpaper glued to the back so that they will stick on the board.

Lettering

Letters being displayed should be at least 2-inches in height. When using letters to convey a message, remember these tips:

- Make it **bold**.
- Make it big so all can see.
- Make it simple.

THREE-DIMENSIONAL VISUAL AIDS

Educators can make use of a wide variety of three-dimensional aids, including:

- Cutout, cutaway, or cross-sectional models
- Working models
- Enlarged models
- Reduced models
- Transparent models
- Fantasized characters or dress (puppets, etc.)

Audiovisual Aids

These include:

- Videocassette tapes
- Slides shows or educational films
- CDs, records, or tapes

All programs, tapes, or recordings should always be previewed before use. After presenting an audiovisual program, the educator should follow up with a discussion that stresses important points and reinforces learning.

Creative Play or Games

This educational strategy is one of the most effective instruments of human understanding and interaction. Children especially enjoy the opportunity to act in plays and dramatizations of stories or events. Several such games and short plays are presented in several sections of this book.

CONSTRUCTING A LARGE TOOTH MODEL

Supplies

12- × 9- × 1-inch piece of Styrofoam (for teeth)
12- × 4.5- × 1-inch piece of Styrofoam (for gums)
Square of white felt
Half square of pink felt
Small pieces of red and black felt (for gingivitis and cavity)
Yarn (for floss)
Yellow or green cotton balls (for plaque)
Six, 2-inch nails
Glue and glue gun

Directions

1. Trace the tooth pattern from Figure 3–1A on the white felt.
2. Trace the gums pattern from Figure 3–1B on the pink felt.
3. Trace the tooth and the gum patterns onto the Styrofoam boards.
4. Cut out the Styrofoam using a serrated knife.
5. Glue the white felt to the Styrofoam teeth to crate the tooth model. Let set.
6. Cut three, 1-inch wide by 4-inch-long strips to use as a divider. Glue one strip on either side, and one in the middle of the Styrofoam teeth.
7. Glue the Styrofoam gums over the three dividers.
8. Dip the nails in glue. Push them from the back of model through the divider pieces and into the gums.
9. Glue the pink felt onto the Styrofoam gums.
10. Cut out red felt for the gums.
11. Cut out black felt for the cavity, following the pattern in Figure 3–1B.
12. Use the colored cotton balls for plaque.

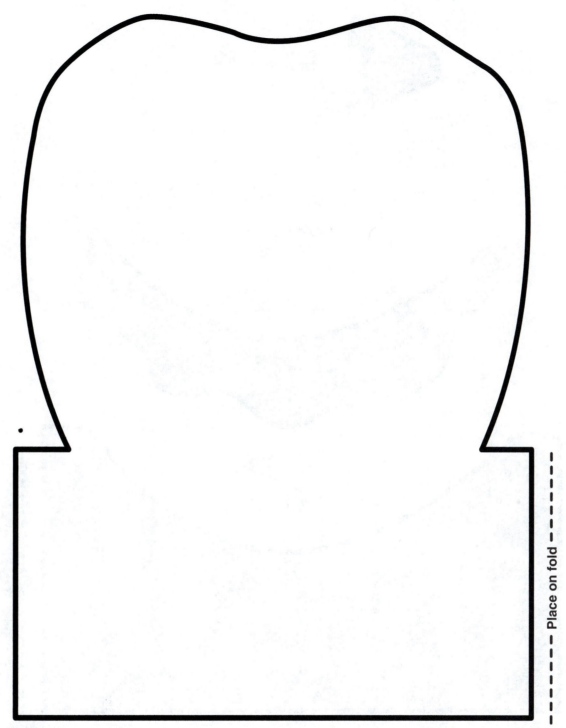

FIGURE 3–1A Large Tooth Pattern.

Place on fold

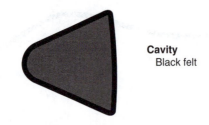

Cavity
Black felt

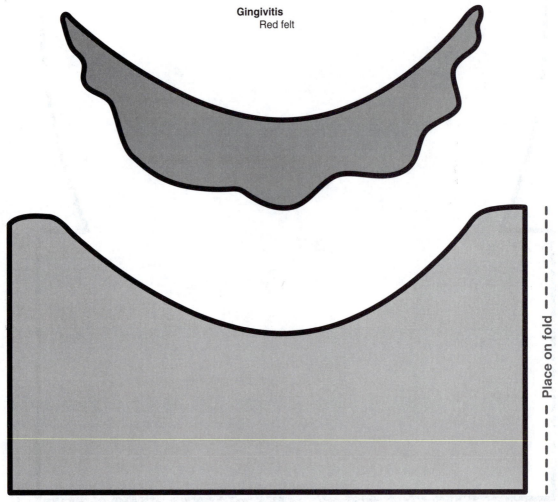

Gingivitis
Red felt

Place on fold

FIGURE 3–1B Large Tooth Pattern.

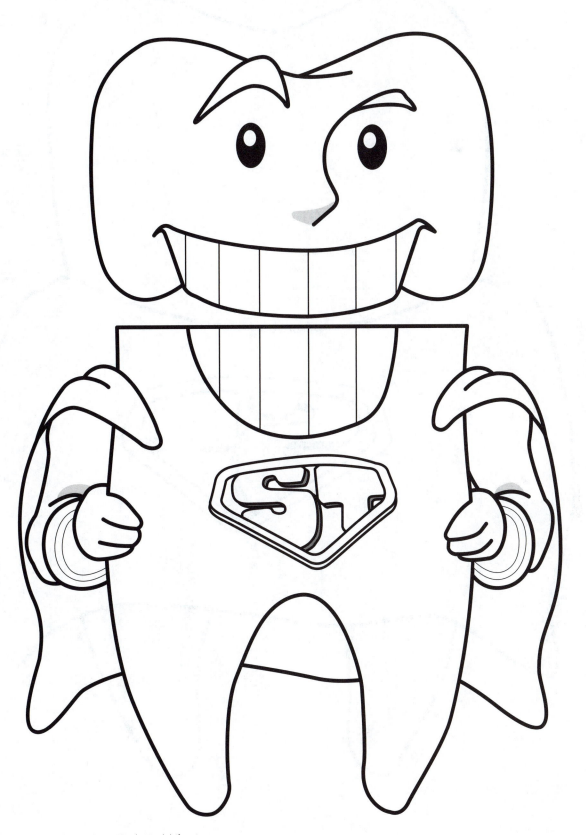

FIGURE 3–2A Super Tooth Model (front).

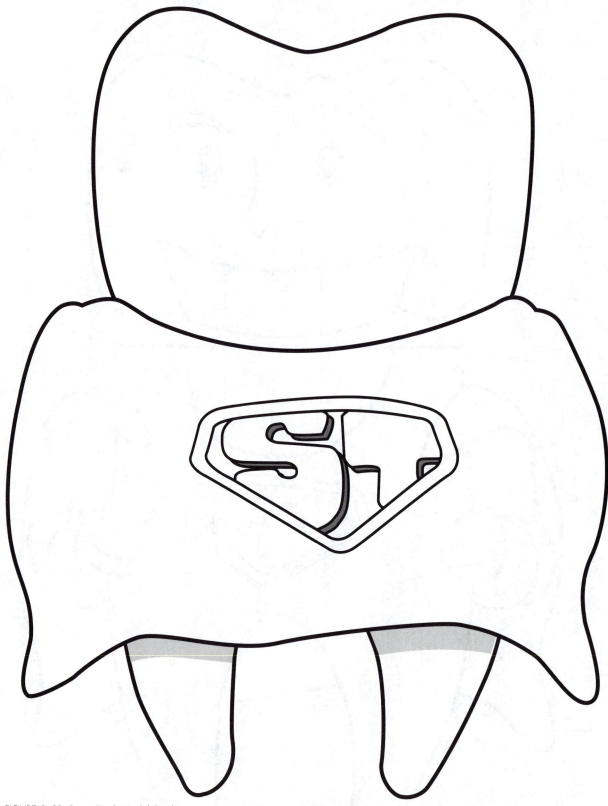

FIGURE 3–2B Super Tooth Model (back).

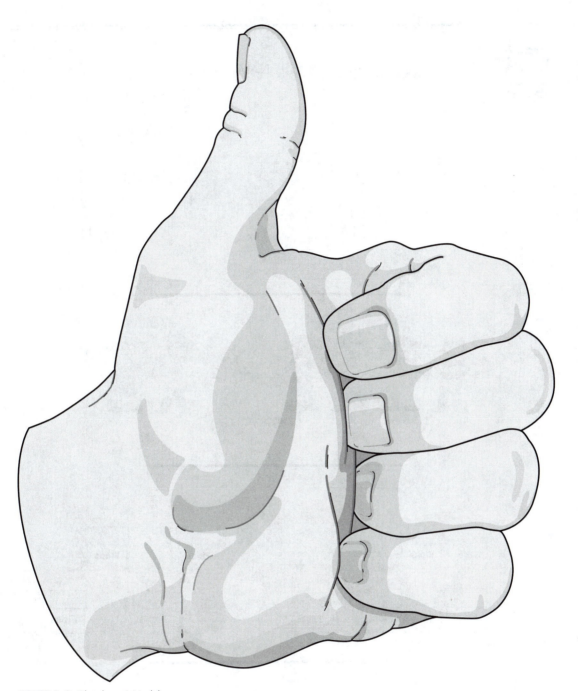

FIGURE 3–3 "Thumbs-up" Model.

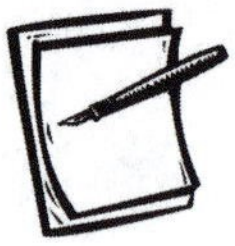

Tooth Math   NAME _____

1. 3 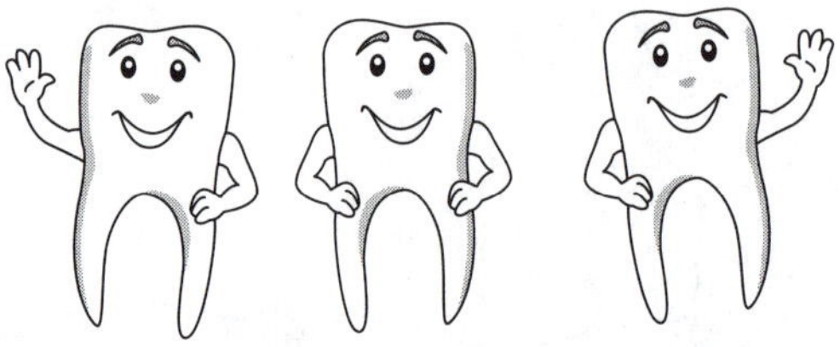 + 1

    = _____

2. 4 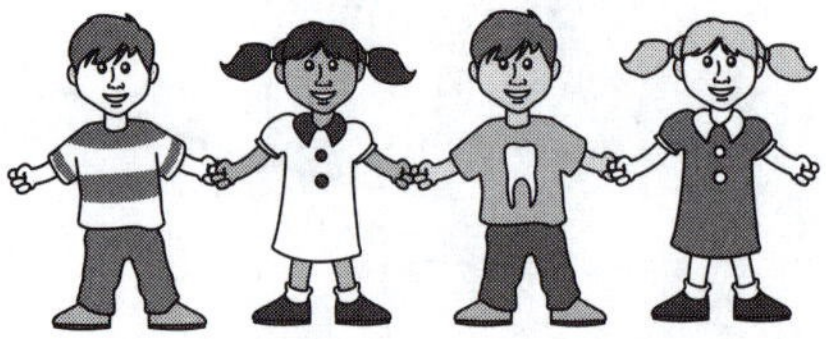 + 2

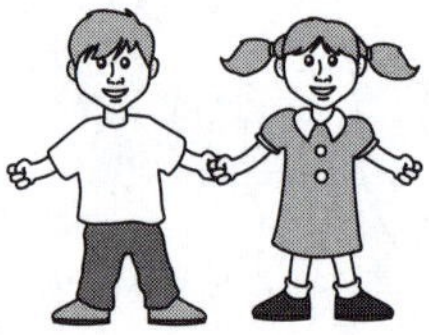

    = _____

3. 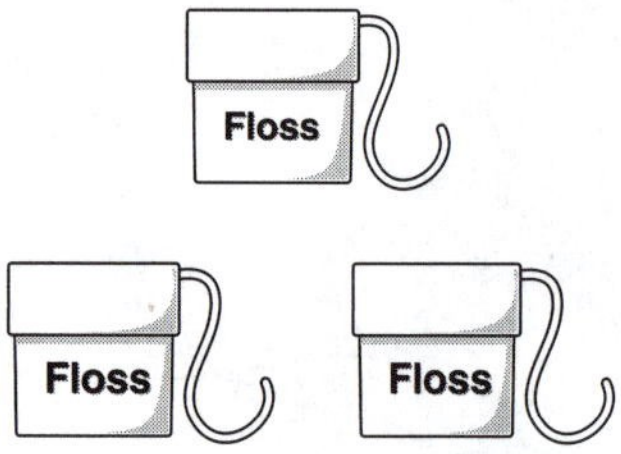 +

    = _____

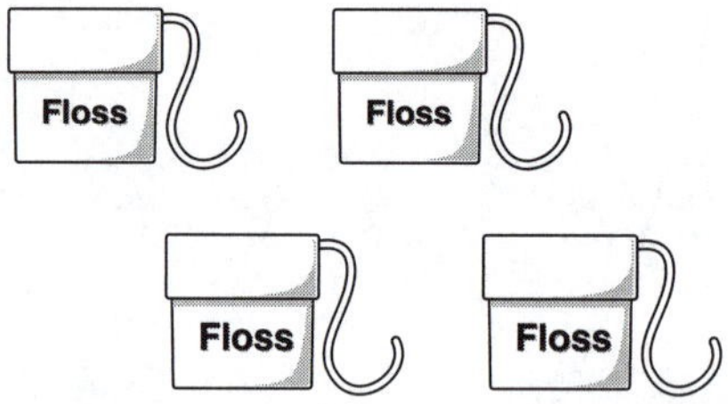

4. How many teeth have you lost?_____Ask your
    neighbor how many teeth they have lost. What is the total
    number of teeth lost?_____.

5. Mary had 8 front teeth. 2 fell out. How many were left?_____

FIGURE 3–4 Tooth Math.

Planning and Implementing a Dental Health

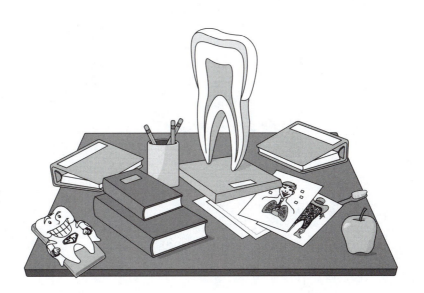

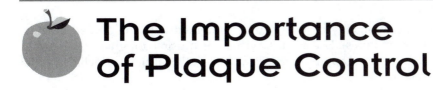

CHAPTER 4

The Importance of Plaque Control

PREPARATION

(5 minutes before beginning lesson)

Assemble the necessary supplies, including disclosing solution or tablets; paper cups; cotton-tipped applicators; small, compact mirrors; and toothbrushes. If appropriate, select students from the class to volunteer for an experiment in which you use a disclosing solution to make the plaque visible.

ANTICIPATORY PLANNING

(5 minutes)

- Review the previous lesson, if applicable.
- Introduce presenters.
- Describe the goals of today's lesson, the format of information, or general topics to be covered.
- Review classroom rules (K–3), if applicable.

General Objectives by Grade Level

(2–3 minutes)

State specifically not more than three objectives appropriate for the classroom learning level that indicate what the majority of the students will be able to achieve by the completion of the lesson. Keep in mind that for every grade level you advance, the previous grade level objectives could also be used.

Upon completion of this lesson, the student will be able to achieve the objectives listed in the following table.

GR	OBJECTIVE
K	Identify that plaque is not pleasant to look at and is not good to have.
	State that plaque can be disturbed with a soft toothbrush.
1	Describe the dental disease process.
	Identify where the plaque hides.
	Identify two consequences of plaque (plaque can hurt your teeth and gums).
	Define plaque and explain its role in the dental disease process.
2	Identify oral disorders caused by plaque accumulations.
3	List warning signs of gum disease.
4	Include any or all of the above information.
5	Include any or all of the above information.
6	Include any or all of the above information.

INSTRUCTION/INFORMATION

(10 minutes)

More than one topic may be included or combined with the guided practice segment (10–20 minutes). Use as many visuals as possible for grades K–3; group discussion may be more appropriate for grades 4–6. Visual aids are included at the end of the lesson.

- Explain the dental disease process.
- Discuss the consequence of leaving plaque on the teeth and gums.
- Relate the story of The Three Friends.

DENTAL DISEASE PROCESS

Show the visual of the dental disease process (Figure 4-1). Discuss how:

Plaque + Sugar = Acid,

Acid + Healthy Tooth = Decay (cavities).

Ask why it is important to brush and floss everyday. (Answer: To remove the plaque that builds up on tooth surfaces.) If the plaque is not removed daily, what can happen? (Discuss.) What are the consequences of leaving plaque on the teeth? (Discuss.) Acid attacks occur every 20 minutes if the plaque is not removed (Discuss).

Discussion/Visual: Related Topics

Discuss the following topics, using additional visuals that you compile or create:

- Bad breath
- Tooth decay (cavities)
- Gum disease (gingivitis); inflammation around the gums

Three Friends Story

The Three Friends

(Developed by the Sacramento County Health Department)

Once upon a time there were three friends. They were sad because they were not like everyone else. Something was missing (see Figure 4-2). What were they missing? (Answer: teeth, mouth, smiles.) Every day they wished they could have teeth and be like everyone else.

One day a good fairy appeared. She said, "I will grant you your wish, but first you must tell me why you want teeth." The first friend said, "I want teeth to help me talk." The second friend said, "I want teeth to help me eat good healthy foods." The third one said, "I want teeth to help me smile."

The good fairy clapped her hands and gave each of them teeth. She told them they were very smart, but they had to promise to brush their teeth everyday to keep them healthy. The three friends promised they would brush daily, and off they went to school.

As the days passed, they had a good time eating, talking, and smiling . . . but they forgot to brush. Then one day the friends noticed that their teeth were getting a yellow film on them and their mouths did not smell very good. The first friend was starting to have pain in one tooth. The three friends asked the school nurse why the tooth hurt, and she told them about plaque:

- Plaque is a bacteria made up of germs found on our teeth.
- Plaque can be invisible or yellow.
- Plaque likes to hide on chewing surfaces, between the teeth, along the gums, and on the tongue.

- Plaque germs like to eat sugar. When they eat sugar, they form acid.
- This acid can make holes in our teeth called cavities.
- Plaque also makes gums red and puffy, and they may bleed.
- People can protect their teeth and keep them healthy by using fluoride, brushing, flossing, eating healthy foods, and going to the dentist.

Now the three friends knew why they needed to take care of their teeth, and they started doing it everyday. They went to their new friend, the dentist, who fixed the hole in the first friend's tooth by filling it with silver. Then they saw the dental hygienist, who cleaned their teeth and put fluoride on them.

By brushing their teeth everyday, their mouths looked, smelled, and felt clean and fresh.

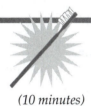

Guided Practice Activities

(10 minutes)

This segment may be combined with the preceding instruction/information segment. Visual aids are included at the end of the lesson.

- Have the students draw a picture of plaque attacking a tooth (see handout).
- Show students how to disclose the plaque.
- Record the number of teeth that are plaque free.
- Remove the plaque by brushing and/or brushing and flossing.

MAKE THE PLAQUE VISIBLE

Preparation

- State exactly what is going to take place using vocabulary appropriate for the grade level (e.g., first grade—"color the plaque"; fourth grade—"use a special disclosing solution"). Emphasize that this experiment will make the plaque visible. You may have the entire class disclose or only a few volunteers. However, this lesson is more effective when everyone discloses, including the teacher(s).
- Outline the steps you will be using on the black/white board: (1) disclose, (2) find the plaque, (3) brush and floss, (4) final check, and (5) rinse brush.

General Rules

- Do not rinse or drink water until you are told to.
- It is not necessary to look at your friends' plaque to improve your own brushing technique.
- Everyone should remain seated throughout the activity.

Using the Disclosing Solution

1. Dispense the disclosing solution on the students' teeth or hand out tablets that can be chewed by each student, as appropriate to the grade level (see below).
   a. *Grades K–2:* Place a small amount of disclosing solution in a paper cup. Use a cotton-tipped applicator to paint the disclosing solution on the students' teeth.
   b. *Grades 3–6:* Have the students line up. Place a small amount of disclosing solution on their tongues and have them swish the solution around in their mouths. (Have them return to their seats to evaluate the plaque.)

2. Pass out small, compact mirrors for the students to use to see where the plaque hides, especially in between the teeth. (Be sure to collect the mirrors at the end of the lesson.)
3. Record the number of teeth that are plaque free.

Removing the Plaque

1. Review the dry brushing and flossing (if applicable) technique to be used.
2. Check to see if the plaque is being removed.
3. Rinse the disclosing solution from the toothbrushes.

Advantages of Using Disclosing Solution

- Students and teachers realize plaque is not some obscure thing that dental personnel talk about.
- They see that they are not doing a thorough job of brushing and are motivated to brush better and more often as a result.
- They see that dry brushing is effective in removing plaque.
- This activity gives you an opportunity to identify cases of gross dental neglect.

Closure

(2–3 minutes)

- Restate the objectives in question form.
- Check students' knowledge and understanding of the concepts presented.
- If time permits, address any other questions the students may have.
- Mention that disclosing solution or tablets can be obtained at their local drug store.

Follow-up Activity

Have students make an "Acid Attack Chart" that lists every snack or meal eaten during the day. Add up the 20-minute periods after each snack or meal to get a total, indicating the amount of time acid is attacking their teeth.

Lesson Plan / PLAQUE CONTROL

Anticipatory Set

Review the previous lesson, if applicable.

Describe goals of today's lesson.

Objectives

1. Describe what plaque is and where it hides.
2. Describe how plaque can be removed.
3. Describe what happens if the plaque is not removed.

Instructions

Show pictures of healthy gums and unhealthy gums and teeth.

Show pictures of the dental disease process.

Relate the story of the three friends, use or enlarge the picture provided at the end of the chapter.

Guided Practice Activities

Question and answer discussion on plaque control and healthy teeth.

Closure

State the above objectives in question form.

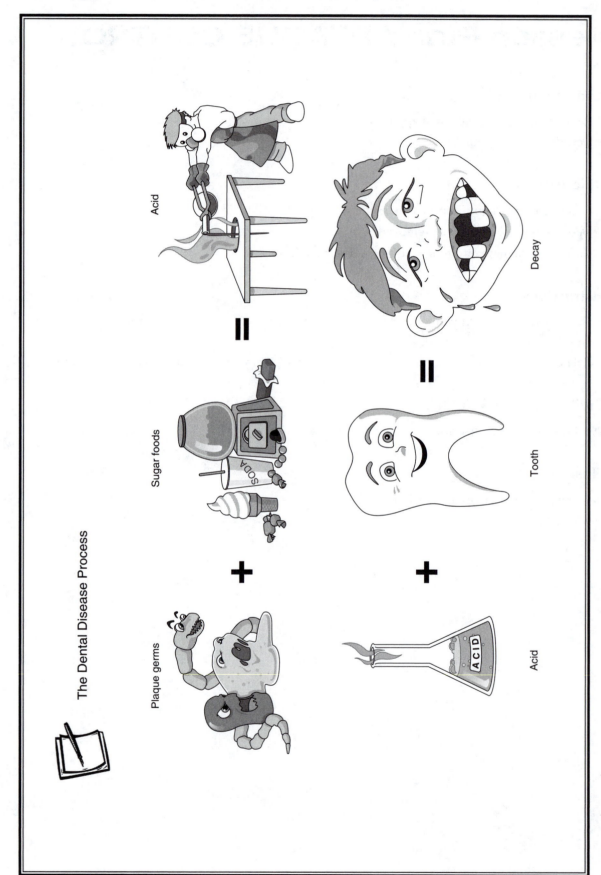

The Dental Disease Process

Plaque germs + Sugar foods = Acid

Tooth + Acid = Decay

Three Friends

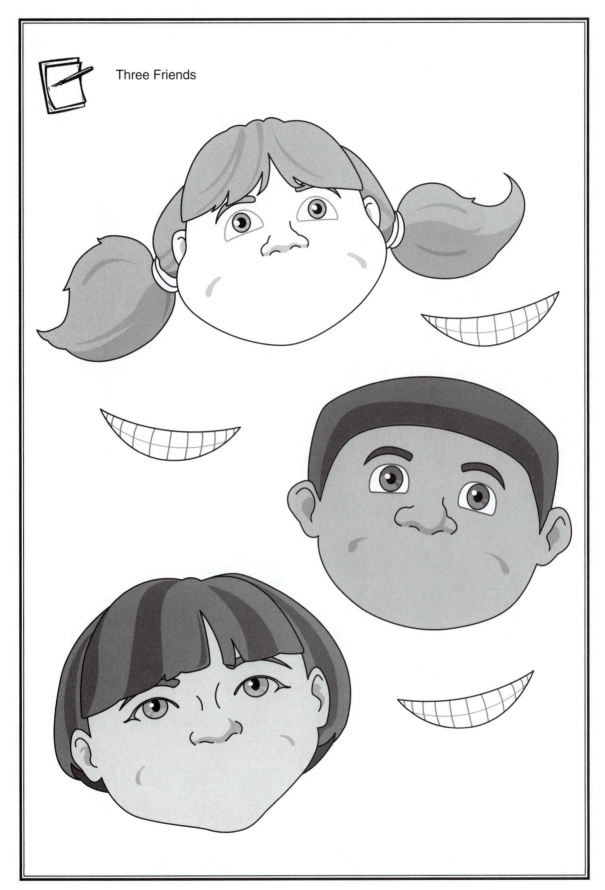

FIGURE 4-2 The Three Friends.

CHAPTER 5

Brushing for Good Oral Health

PREPARATION

(5 minutes)

Large toothbrush and model, display a variety of toothbrushes; include some with poor bristles, good bristles, soft and hard, different style toothbrush handles and lengths, etc., for discussion.

ANTICIPATORY SET

- Review the previous lesson if applicable.
- Introduce presenters.
- Describe the goals of today's lesson, the format of information, and general topics to be covered.
- Review classroom rules (K–3), if applicable.

General Objectives by Grade Level

(2–3 minutes)

State specifically not more than three objectives appropriate for the classroom learning level that indicate what the majority of the students will be able to achieve by the completion of the lesson. This lesson may also be incorporated with the objectives and information from the toothbrushing and plaque control lesson. Keep in mind that for every grade level you advance, the previous grade level objectives could also be used.

Upon completion of this lesson, the student will be able to achieve the objectives listed in the following table.

GR	OBJECTIVE
K	Describe plaque.
	Describe how plaque can hurt teeth and gums, and areas where plaque hides.
	State the consequences of too much plaque in the mouth.
1	List the characteristics of a good toothbrush and storage recommendations.
2	Demonstrate increased proficiency in brushing teeth.
3	Explain the process of decay, and tell why regular dental visits are important for diagnosing dental problems at their earliest stages.
4	Discuss the signs and causes of periodontal disease, and relate the effects of proper brushing to maintaining the health of the gingiva.
	Discuss the importance to oral health of both personal and professional care.
5	Relate the results of dental neglect to decay and periodontal disease.
	Recognize that each person is responsible for his or her own dental health.
6	Include any or all of the above information.

INSTRUCTION/INFORMATION

(10 minutes)

More than one topic may be included or combined with the guided practice segment (10–20 minutes). Use as many visuals as possible for grades K–3; group discussion may be more appropriate for grades 4–6.

- Discuss plaque (see the previous lesson).
- Explain how brushing daily removes the plaque.

Plaque and Your Teeth

Discussion/Visual: What Is Plaque?

Plaque is a sticky, clear substance that forms on teeth. It is made of germs and is not good for your teeth. Plaque forms on the teeth every time you eat. If it is not removed, it causes dental diseases. Plaque hides along the gum line (sulcus), in between teeth, and on every surface of the tooth. If plaque is not removed along the gum line, it causes gingivitis (red, puffy gums). If plaque is not removed on the tooth surfaces, it creates acids that eat into the tooth surface, causing cavities (holes in the teeth).

Use visuals to present the following dental disease equations (see the earlier plaque control lesson; Figure 4-1 for tooth decay and gum disease):

Plaque (germs) + Sugar (from the foods we eat) = Acid,

Acid + Healthy Tooth = Decay (hole in the tooth),

Plaque (germs) + Sugar (from the foods we eat) = Toxin,

Toxin + Healthy Gums = Gingivitis (red, puffy gums; gum disease).

Discussion/Visual: Removing the Plaque

Discuss the variety of different types and sizes of toothbrushes that are available. Emphasize the following points:

- Plaque must be removed daily.
- Brush your teeth at least twice a day.
- The most important time to brush is after meals and before going to bed.
- Be sure your toothbrush bristles are soft, straight, and firm. Discard your toothbrush when the bristles become frayed and worn.
- Be sure your toothbrush is the right size for your mouth.
- Never share your toothbrush.

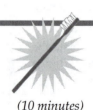

Guided Practice Activities

(10 minutes)

This segment may be combined with the preceding instruction/information segment. Visual aids are included at the end of the lesson.

- Illustrate the dry toothbrushing technique in the classroom. Emphasize that toothpaste gives the teeth fluoride protection, but it is not needed to remove the plaque.

CLASSROOM BRUSHING

Preliminary Demonstration/Discussion

Use Figures 5-1–5-3 for assistance.

1. Demonstrate the proper way to hold a toothbrush.
2. Demonstrate a short, back-and-forth, systematic brushing motion.
3. Describe a sequence for brushing all tooth surfaces.
4. Demonstrate brushing the tongue.
5. Demonstrate proper care of the toothbrush.

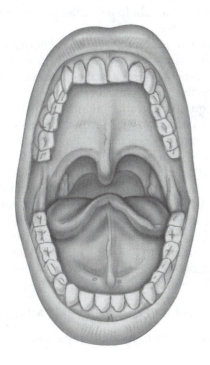

FIGURE 5–1 The Mouth

Preparation

- Put students' names on (toothbrush handles).
- Provide toothbrush holders that students can keep at their desks.

General Rules for Brushing

- There should be a toothbrush for each person. Never use anyone else's toothbrush and never allow anyone else to use yours.
- Keep your toothbrush clean. Rinse it under cold running water after brushing. Shake out the excess water and replace it in the holder to air dry.
- Do not store brushes in their original wrappers (box or plastic).
- Replace your toothbrush when it becomes badly worn (every few months), or when bristles are frayed or falling out. Never chew on your brush. A brush that is used properly will last much longer than one that is mistreated.
- Never walk around the room with a toothbrush in your mouth. Always carry your brush in your hand to prevent injuries to your mouth that might occur from accidental falls or getting bumped while the toothbrush is in your mouth.
- Brush your teeth at least twice a day, especially before bedtime.

Initial Brushing Session

1. Using your own brush, demonstrate the proper way to hold a toothbrush.
   a. Grasp the toothbrush with the entire hand, with the thumb pointing toward the bristles.
   b. Use a firm grasp.
2. Pass out the toothbrushes.
3. Have the students demonstrate the proper way to hold the toothbrush.
   a. Have the students hold the toothbrush high in the air.
   b. Quickly check each student.
4. Demonstrate the short, back-and-forth brushing motion outside the mouth.
5. Have each student hold his or her toothbrush in the air and practice moving it in short strokes.
6. Explain the importance of brushing both the teeth and the gums; that is, the toothbrush is placed where the teeth and gums come together. Have students vibrate the bristles of their brushes in place.
7. Have the students demonstrate their proficiency in brushing by dry brushing one quadrant in their mouths. Quickly check each student's technique, watching particularly for proper placement of the toothbrush.
8. When proficiency is achieved, have students brush all quadrants, starting in the outside upper right and moving to the upper left, and then the outside lower left to lower right; then brushing from the inside upper right to upper left; and finally, from the inside lower left to lower right.
   a. Check for the shortness and direction of the stroke.
   b. Have students brush the biting surfaces and tongue.
9. Emphasize the importance of systematic brushing so no areas are missed.
10. Instruct students to allow the toothbrush to air dry before putting it away.
11. Tell students to repeat this activity at least twice a day (average brushing time is 2–4 minutes).

TOOTHBRUSH STORAGE CONTAINERS

Show several different types of storage containers for toothbrushes. Emphasize the following points:

- Always let the toothbrush air dry before putting it away.
- Be sure the container is clearly marked with your name.
- Never store a toothbrush in a plastic wrapper.

CLOSURE

(2–3 minutes)

- Restate the objectives in question form.
- Check students' knowledge and understanding of the concepts presented.
- If time permits, address any other questions the students may have.

Lesson Plan / TOOTHBRUSHING

Anticipatory Set

Review the previous lesson if applicable.

Describe the goals of the today's lesson.

Objectives

Describe the proper motion for toothbrushing.

Demonstrate effective plaque removal with toothbrushing.

Describe the qualities of a good toothbrush.

Instructions

Discuss various types, style and qualities of toothbrushes.

Discuss and demonstrate the proper and effective way to remove plaque.

Show pictures with good tooth brushes/bad tooth brushes, plaque removal etc.

Guided Practice Activities

Establish a pattern for brush, look at hand positioning for brushing.

Practice brushing at home or in the classroom.

Closure

Restate the objectives in question form.

Brushing

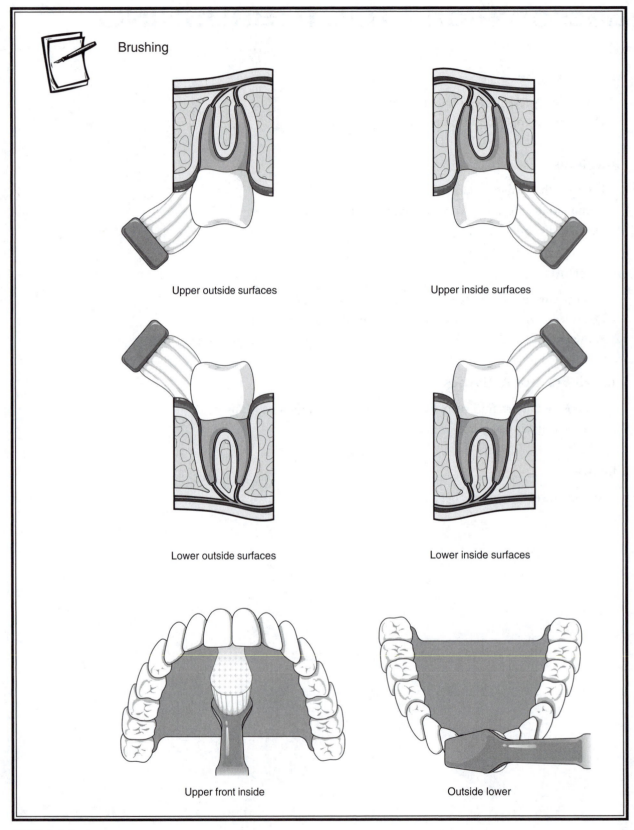

Upper outside surfaces

Upper inside surfaces

Lower outside surfaces

Lower inside surfaces

Upper front inside

Outside lower

FIGURE 5–2 Brushing.

Pattern of Brushing

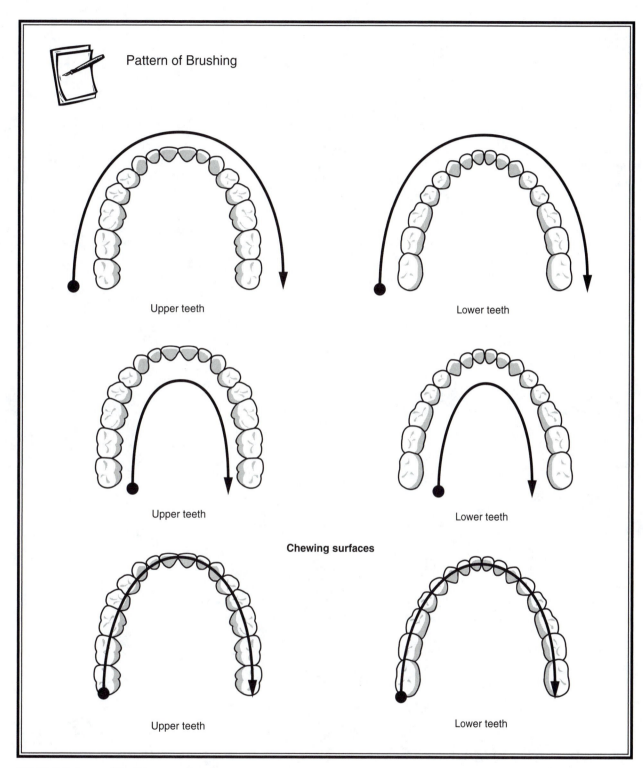

Upper teeth   Lower teeth

Upper teeth   Lower teeth

Chewing surfaces

Upper teeth   Lower teeth

FIGURE 5–3 Pattern of Brushing.

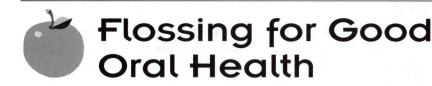

CHAPTER 6

Flossing for Good Oral Health

PREPARATION

(5 minutes before beginning lesson)

Assemble the following items: several different samples of floss (tape, waxed, unwaxed, flavored, fluoride) and a large picture of the mouth. Use Figures 6-1 and 6-2 for assistance.

ANTICIPATORY PLANNING

(5 minutes)

- Review the previous lesson if applicable.
- Introduce presenters.
- Describe the goals of today's lesson, the format of information, or general topics to be covered.
- Review classroom rules (K–3), if applicable.
- Review the dental disease process (see Figure 4-1).
- Reiterate that toothbrushing does not remove plaque between the teeth.

General Objectives by Grade Level

(2–3 minutes)

State specifically not more than three objectives appropriate for the classroom learning level that indicate what the majority of the students will be able to achieve by the completion of the lesson. Keep in mind that for every grade level you advance, the previous grade level objectives could also be used.

Upon completion of this lesson, the student will be able to achieve the objectives listed in the following table.

GR	OBJECTIVE
K	Identify dental floss.
1	Describe the function of floss.
2	Explain the importance of floss following an activity that demonstrates its use.
	Relate the lack of interproximal decay and gingival irritation (redness or bleeding) to daily flossing.
3	Demonstrate the ability to floss both front (mesial) and back (distal) sides of the teeth throughout the mouth.
	Identify the gingival sulcus and show how to use dental floss to keep this area clean.
	Demonstrate the use of floss in all areas of the mouth with and without the use of a floss holder.
4	Include any or all of the above information.
5	Include any or all of the above information.
6	Include any or all of the above information.

INSTRUCTION/INFORMATION

(10 minutes)

More than one topic may be included or combined with the guided practice segment (10–20 minutes). Use as many visuals as possible for grades K–3; group discussion may be more appropriate for grades 4–6.

- Discuss the importance of daily flossing.
- Describe the different types of floss available.
- Describe the floss holder (see Figure 14-3).

General Information

First, ask students how they might remove plaque from between the teeth. Explain how the brush would not fit there. Ask students: (1) if they have tried flossing before, and (2) how many have floss in their home or have seen their parents floss.

Explain the different types of floss available: tape, waxed, unwaxed, flavored (colored), fluoride, and floss holders (Figure 14-3). Show samples of each. Demonstrate flossing technique by using real floss on your own front teeth.

Guided Practice Activities

(10 minutes)

This segment may be combined with the preceding instruction/information segment. Visual aids are included at the end of the lesson.

- Relate the story of The Big King.
- Perform the yarn activity for grades K–2.
- Do the Flossing Big Teeth activity for grades 1–3.
- Demonstrate flossing in the classroom for grades 3–6.

**Flossing
Story**

The Big King

To be told after flossing is taught and before practice to reinforce flossing concepts.

Make two tooth costumes. Using a white pillow case, draw a large happy molar on one side and a sad molar on the other (see Figure 6-4). Provide prince and princess crowns and a toothbrush.

Once upon a time in a faraway land, there lived a great BIG king who had great BIG teeth. The king lived in a great BIG palace and had many servants. One day the king was looking at his teeth and saw lots of plaque. There was plaque on the sides of his teeth and even in between. The king was really sad; the teeth were sad, too! *(Why?)*

The king wanted his teeth clean, but he did not know how to clean them. He called out, "Servants! Servants! Come clean my teeth." The servants could not believe the king would ask such a thing. They all agreed to say no to the king. They said, "No way! We clean the floors; we clean the windows; we make the food. We will not clean your teeth, too!" This made the king angry, and he told the servants, "You are all fired! Go home!" Now the king was all alone, and he still did not know how to clean his teeth. He sat and thought and thought until he fell fast asleep (zzzzz!).

In the middle of the night, along came a fairy princess. (Pick a girl from the class to be the princess; give her a crown and a toothbrush.) The princess thought that maybe if she brushed the plaque away, the king might call the servants back to the palace, and the king and his teeth would be happy. However, there was one place her brush would not fit. Does anyone know where that was? (*In between*).

The princess was not easily discouraged. She called on her friend, who was a prince. (Pick a boy from the class to be the prince; give him a crown and yarn for floss.) He had a very special piece of string. What is the name of this special string? (*Dental floss*). The prince moved the floss up and down, resting it on the side of the king's teeth, to remove the plaque. He flossed all of the king's teeth—front teeth, molars, on top, and on the bottom.

The prince and princess were all done, and just in time—the king was about to wake up. The king opened his eyes and called out, "Where's my breakfast?" Then he remembered that he was all alone. Just at that moment, he looked at his teeth and saw that they were sparkling clean. That made the king so happy, do you know what he did? He called all the servants back to the palace that day and said, "Today you will all have fun. Nobody works today."

The king thought that the servants cleaned his teeth. Let us not tell him, okay? Because the servants, the prince, and princess, the king, and his teeth all lived happily ever after.

Follow-up Activity for The Big King

Have students in grades 3–6 practice flossing. Supplement with the yarn activity for grades K–2.

Guided Practice Activities

FLOSSING YARN ACTIVITY (FOR GRADES K–2)

Directions

1. Cut pieces of yarn that are approximately 12 inches long and pass them out to all students.
2. Explain the purpose of flossing, demonstrate flossing, and show students real dental floss.
3. Introduce the activity by telling students that the yarn will represent floss and their fingers, teeth.
4. Model the activity first by having one adult demonstrate flossing on a hand (representing five teeth).

Winding the "Floss"

1. Instruct students to hold the "floss" like a bicycle handle. They should leave a little "floss" sticking out of each fist.
2. Have them point two index fingers straight out, then to the floor, then toward themselves, then to the ceiling. Have them pinch the "floss" with their index finger and thumb.
3. Tell students to "floss" carefully on both sides of their partner's "teeth" (fingers). They should floss one hand first, then the other.

Do not begin the activity until each partner has a piece of floss. Talk the students through the winding and flossing, and when the students are finished flossing both of their partner's hands, have them hold their floss up high. When all are ready (all hands are raised with floss), instruct the students to exchange roles.

FLOSSING BIG TEETH (FOR GRADES 1–3 AND SPECIAL EDUCATION)

Anticipatory Set

Educator flosses own teeth in front of the classroom. When ready to begin lesson, the instructor ask the class what he or she is doing and why.

Objectives

By the end of the lesson the participant will be able to:

1. Explain the importance of daily flossing.
2. Identify the incisors, cuspids, bicuspids, and molars, and describe their functions.

Instruction

Flossing is demonstrated on large tooth model using yarn (floss) and cotton balls (green or yellow represents plaque). Talk about the types of floss and have examples of wax, unwaxed, colored, etc. Pass around floss samples for the participants to look at, feel, and smell (flavored).

Four participants (volunteers) come forward to represent the four types of teeth. A large cutout of each of the following teeth is held by the four students: incisor, cuspid, bicuspid, and molar. (Use Figure 6-2 for assistance cutout can have string attached to wear around the participant's neck.)

Have the students stand very close together, then place the cotton balls in between the students who are representing the teeth. Explain that the plaque sticks in between the teeth, just as the cotton balls stick in between the standing students. Ask another student to take a large piece of yarn and wrap it around his or her fingers (educators may need to help the student). The student should floss between the teeth (students standing together), removing all the plaque.

Write the names of the teeth and their functions on the board. Use Figure 6-3 and Figure 12.2 for assistance:

$$INCISOR = CUT$$

Floss holders: detailed information about the use of floss holders can be found on page 139 if you could like to include this information as well.

Guided Practice

Floss finger activity or use of real floss in the anterior teeth to start off with; move to the posterior if participants show coordination and willingness to continue.

Closure

Participants are questioned about the purpose and frequency of flossing, the types of floss to use, and the names of the teeth and their functions. For upper grades, discuss the number of each type of tooth found in the mouth. For example, there are 8 incisors (4 on the top and 4 on the bottom) and 4 cuspids (2 on the top and 2 on the bottom etc.).

Independent Practice

Encourage students to floss daily at home with parental help or supervision.

FINGER FLOSSING (FOR GRADES 3–6)

(Use Figure 6-1 for assistance.)

Finger Flossing

Dental floss helps get your teeth really clean by removing plaque from between your teeth and under the gums.

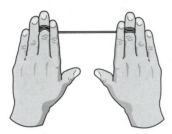

1. Wrap about 18 inches of floss around your middle fingers.

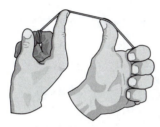

3. Use your thumb and index finger to guide the floss between your upper teeth.

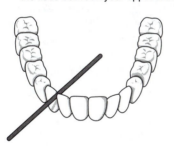

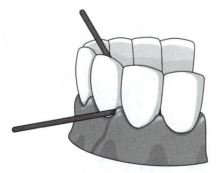

7. Now pull the floss against the tooth. Move the floss gently under the gum until you feel resistance. Move to a clean area of floss after every two or three teeth.

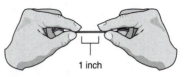

1 inch

2. "Pinch on inch" of floss.

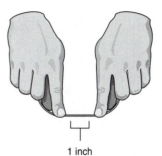

1 inch

4. Use your index fingers to guide the floss between your lower teeth.

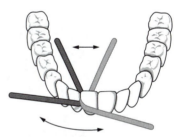

6. Bend the floss around the tooth in a C or U shape.

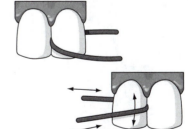

8. Holding the floss firmly against your tooth, scrape the plaque from the side of your tooth, moving the floss up and down five times. Be sure to floss both sides of each tooth.

Move to a clean area of floss after every two or three teeth.

FIGURE 6-1 Finger Flossing

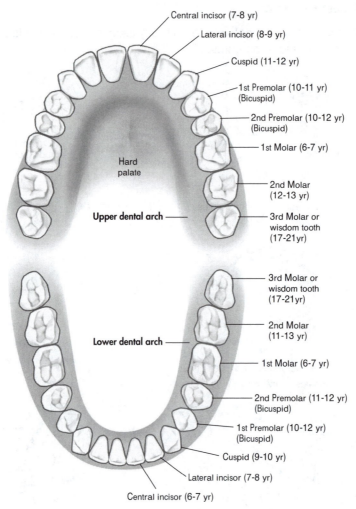

Central incisor (7-8 yr)

Lateral incisor (8-9 yr)

Cuspid (11-12 yr)

1st Premolar (10-11 yr)
(Bicuspid)

2nd Premolar (10-12 yr)
(Bicuspid)

1st Molar (6-7 yr)

Hard palate

2nd Molar
(12-13 yr)

Upper dental arch

3rd Molar or
wisdom tooth
(17-21yr)

3rd Molar or
wisdom tooth
(17-21yr)

2nd Molar
(11-13 yr)

Lower dental arch

1st Molar (6-7 yr)

2nd Premolar (11-12 yr)
(Bicuspid)

1st Premolar (10-12 yr)
(Bicuspid)

Cuspid (9-10 yr)

Lateral incisor (7-8 yr)

Central incisor (6-7 yr)

FIGURE 6–2 The Teeth.

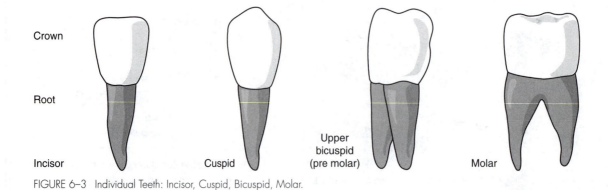

Crown

Root

Incisor

Cuspid

Upper
bicuspid
(pre molar)

Molar

FIGURE 6–3 Individual Teeth: Incisor, Cuspid, Bicuspid, Molar.

Preliminary Demonstration/Discussion

1. Demonstrate flossing on yourself; use finger exercise again.
2. Measure and tear off floss from individual containers and pass out to students. Pieces should be about 18 inches long.
3. Explain that when flossing students must be careful not to injure the gums. If they do, they might bleed. (Use the analogy of getting a paper cut.)

General Rules for Flossing

- Do not jam the floss between your teeth.
- Always be in control of the floss.
- To floss your lower teeth, put one finger on the inside of your teeth.
- To floss your upper teeth, put the pointer finger inside to guide the floss.
- Establish a path or journey so that no teeth are missed.
- Be sure to hug the side of the next tooth and slide the floss up and down the side of that tooth.
- Throw the floss away when you are through (2–3 minutes).

CLOSURE

- Restate the objectives in question form.
- Check the students' knowledge and understanding of the concepts presented.
- If time permits, address any other questions the students may have.

Lesson Plan / FLOSSING

Anticipatory Set

Review previous lesson if applicable.

Describe today's lesson.

Review the dental disease process.

Objectives

1. Describe the importance of flossing daily.
2. Describe the different types of floss and floss holders.
3. Demonstrate the ability to floss both the front and back teeth.

Instructions

Discuss the importance of daily flossing, types of floss and floss holders.

Demonstrate flossing procedure.

Relate the story of the Big king.

Guided Practice Activities

If applicable have the student demonstrate flossing.

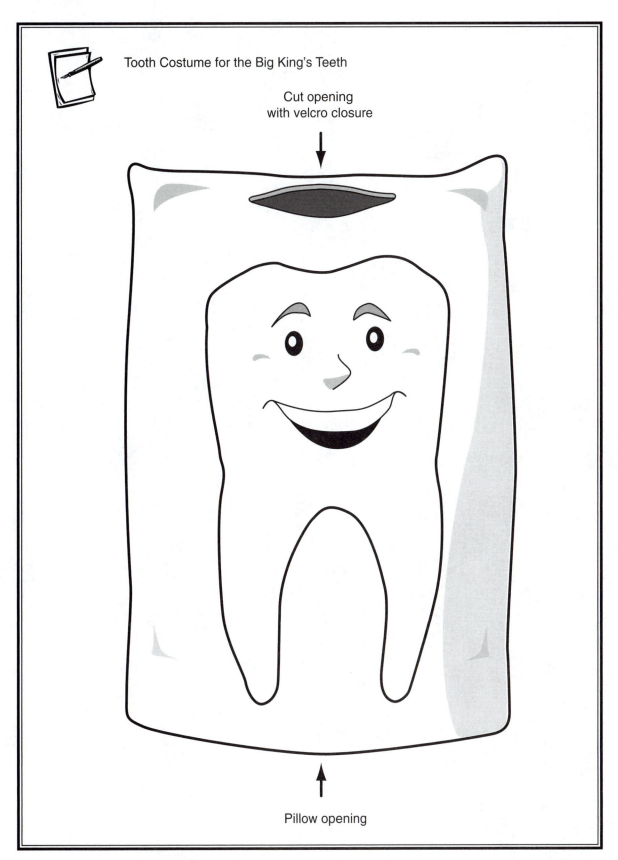

Tooth Costume for the Big King's Teeth

Cut opening
with velcro closure

Pillow opening

FIGURE 6–4 Tooth Costume for the Big King's Teeth.

CHAPTER 7

The Use of Fluoride

PREPARATION

(5 minutes before beginning lesson)

Bring a variety of items or pictures that contain fluoride, such as green leafy vegetables, fish or tuna, vitamins, tablets, toothpaste, mouth rinse, water, and gel for fluoride trays. Write the word "fluoride" on the board. Bring information from your local water department about the addition of fluoride to the public water supply. Use Tables 7-1 and 7-2 for assistance.

ANTICIPATORY PLANNING

(5 minutes)

- Review the previous lesson if applicable.
- Introduce presenters.
- Describe the goals of today's lesson, the format of information, or general topics to be covered.
- Review classroom rules (grades K–3), if applicable.
- Survey the classroom's fluoride exposure. (Ask: "How many of you use toothpaste or drink water with fluoride?")

General Objectives by Grade Level

(2–3 minutes)

State specifically not more than three objectives appropriate for the classroom learning level that indicate what the majority of the students will be able to achieve by the completion of the lesson. Keep in mind for every grade level you advance, the previous grade level objectives could also be used.

Upon completion of this lesson, the student will be able to achieve the objectives listed in the following table.

GR	OBJECTIVES
K	Explain that fluoride contributes to oral health.
1	Describe topical fluoride.
2	Describe the benefits of using fluoride.
3	Name and explain the two types of fluoride (topical and systemic).
4	Describe fluoride sources.
5	Include any or all of the above information.
6	Include any or all of the above information.

INSTRUCTION/INFORMATION

(10 minutes)

More than one topic may be included or combined with the guided practice segment (10–15 minutes). Use as many visual aids as possible for grades K–3; group discussion may be more appropriate for grades 4–6.

- Review the general information; make a chart comparing the two types of fluorides (topical and systemic).
- Emphasize how fluoride contributes to oral health. (Fluoride is a nutrient and a mineral that makes teeth stronger.)
- Utilize discussion: A happy smile begins with fluoridation.
- Present the history of fluoride.

General Information

Fluoride is an essential mineral necessary for proper bone and tooth formation. It is found in trace amounts in most foods and in varying amounts in water. The most effective and inexpensive way to reduce dental decay in a community is through water fluoridation. Because many areas do not have optimal fluoride levels in the water (approximately one part per million), the supplemental use of fluorides has proven extremely effective in the reduction of decay.

A fluoride that is swallowed is called a *systemic fluoride*. It is incorporated into the tooth structure from inside the body. The fluoride ion combines with tooth enamel to make a more perfect crystal (called *hydroxyapatite* or H-5 dental enamel) that is more resistant to decay. Examples of systemic fluorides include fluoridation of city water, fluoride tablets or drops, and very small amounts of fluoride found in foods such as dark green leafy vegetables, fish, and apples.

Fluorides that are exposed directly to the tooth are called *topical fluorides*. Topical fluorides are applied to a tooth after the tooth has erupted into the mouth. Examples of topical fluorides include fluoride toothpaste, mouth rinse, and treatments given by a dentist or dental hygienists or in school fluoride rinse programs.

Fluoride is not the only thing necessary for good dental health, but the protection fluoride gives has been shown to reduce decay from 20 percent to 60 percent, depending on the source, timing, and duration of the fluoride supplement. Fluoride protection in combination with effective plaque removal beginning at an early age and a reduced intake of sweets can contribute to a marked decrease in dental disease over an entire lifetime.

The most effective and inexpensive way to reduce dental decay in a community is through water fluoridation. When water fluoridation cannot be utilized, self-applied fluorides are also effective in reducing decay at a minimal cost. A prescription for 0.2 percent sodium fluoride mouth rinse or 0.25 mg tablet benefits children who do not obtain optimal levels of systemic fluoride. Sodium fluoride mouth rinse has been demonstrated to have several advantages when used in a school-based rinsing program, among them: (1) it takes little time (3–5 minutes a week), (2) it is inexpensive and simple to distribute to the participants, and (3) its use requires limited professional supervision.

For detailed information on fluoride products refer to the appendix.

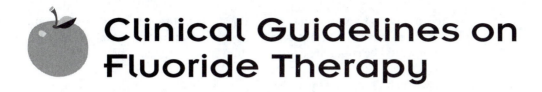

Clinical Guidelines on Fluoride Therapy

AMERICAN ACADEMY OF PEDIATRIC DENTISTRY
(REVISED 2003)

1. Fluoride toothpaste containing the ADA seal of acceptance should be used—a pea-sized amount with each brushing. The dentist or dental hygienist should advise as to number of brushing per day.
2. Children at high risk for dental decay (i.e., children with braces children who have reduced salivary flow, or who are unable to clean teeth properly, or who are at dietary risk, or have mothers or siblings with caries, or have high levels of bacteria that cause cavities) should consider additional fluoride therapy—rinses, gels, or drops. These can be recommended by the dentist or dental hygienist.

First Smiles

Dental Health Begins at Birth (A Project by the California First Five Oral Health Initiative and Collaborative Effort Between The California Dental Association Foundation and The Dental Health Foundation)

1. Daily use of a fluoride toothpaste in the morning and before bedtime should be encouraged for all babies and young children.
2. Fluoride varnish is a highly concentrated fluoride product that can be beneficial for high-risk babies and young children.

DISCUSSION: A HAPPY SMILE BEGINS WITH FLUORIDATION

Topic: Local Water Fluoridation

Visit your local water company. Gather pamphlets, booklets, and other materials pertaining to fluoridation and the water system. Find out how much fluoride is in the local water supply. Is the fluoride natural (from ground water) or added? This lesson is a great way to infuse a dental concept into a science/environment curriculum. Information may also be available on-line.

Topic: Body Systems and Water

Human bodies are made up of 70 percent water. Therefore, every system in the body uses water. Review the following questions:

- Why is water important to our teeth?
- What body system do our teeth belong to?

Topic: Minerals in Water

Water is a solvent. Therefore, many minerals are found in water. Review the following questions:

- What are the two minerals found in water that are important to our teeth and bones? (*Answer*: Fluoride and calcium.)
- Drinking water can be a good source of fluoride. Is your city water fluoridated?
- How much fluoride should you have in your drinking water to prevent tooth decay (cavities)? (*Answer*: Dentists, doctors, and scientists recommend one part per million (ppm). If you live where the weather is warmer, the

recommended amount may be slightly less but never less than 0.7 ppm. This is because in warmer climates, people tend to drink more water. One ppm would be equal to one drop of fluoride in 10 gallons of water.)

Topic: How Much Fluoride Do We Need?

The water from the utilities must be safe for everyone to use. Fluoride is a naturally occurring mineral found in or added to water. Fluoridation has been studied for almost 50 years and has been found to be safe. Fluoride in the drinking water is one of the most cost-effective ways to reduce dental decay. However, just like with vitamins, minerals, or medicine, people need to follow the recommended amount of fluoride. The recommended amount is based on age and how much, if any, fluoride is in the drinking water system (see Tables 7-1 and 7-2.) Additional fluoride information can also be found in the appendix section (page 223–224.)

Fluoride Story

The History of Fluoride (A True Story)

Once upon a time, over 80 years ago, a dentist named Frederick McKay moved to Colorado Springs from the East Coast. Because Dr. McKay was trained as a dentist, he wanted to do just what he had done in the east for a living, that is, to help people have healthy mouths and good gums, and to fix cavities or holes in the teeth of those who had not learned that brushing away plaque and eating less sugary foods would prevent these cavities from forming. He opened his new office and put out his sign, "Dr. Frederick McKay, D.D.S." (Write D.D.S. on the board and explain the abbreviation.)

Dr. McKay hoped people would come to him for help. Soon people did begin to come in for X-rays (which are used to find cavities in between the teeth, and to check formation of permanent teeth in the jaws of younger patients), for checkups, and to have their teeth cleaned. However, one thing soon became clear—almost none of them had decay (holes in their teeth). The only people with cavities were those like Dr. McKay, who had come from out of town.

Dr. McKay and others asked many questions of these patients. They asked about what they ate and what they drank, trying to find out why they did not have a problem with cavities like people from other parts of the country did. It took almost 25 years of asking questions and studying the possibilities to discover that the answer was found in the water the people in Colorado were drinking. The water came from the hills in streams from melting snow and it contained a substance called *fluoride.* (Write the term on the board.)

Let me show you a rock like those from the hills in Colorado above where Dr. McKay lived. (Hold up a rock.) How do you suppose the fluoride found in this rock gets into the water to make teeth strong? As the water passes over the rocks a tiny, tiny bit of fluoride joins the flowing water from the streams and rivers. This is what happened in Dr. McKay's town. Eventually, the water reached the people in Colorado Springs, and they drank this water and the enamel of their teeth got harder and stronger. This was not the very best way to get just the right amount of fluoride, however, because sometimes when the streams were full and running fast there was a different amount of fluoride in the water than in the summer when the water in the streams and rivers was low. After many, many studies and tests, just the right amount of fluoride for water was discovered. One part of fluoride per one million parts of water makes strong teeth that are nice and white.

Many cities have fluoride in their water in this amount, and the people in those cities are fortunate because just by turning on the faucet and drinking water, cooking foods in this water, and brushing their teeth with this water, they will have stronger, harder teeth with fewer cavities.

Table 7–1 Systemic Flouride: Supplemental Fluoride Concentration (ppm) (mg/day) 1994

	Domestic Water Fluoride Dosage Schedule		
Age	*< 0.3 ppm*	*0.3–0.6 ppm*	*> 0.6 ppm*
6 months–3 years	0.25 mg/day	0	0
3–6 years	0.5 mg/day	0.25 mg/day	0
6–16 years	1.0 mg/day	0.5 mg/day	0

ppm = parts per million.

Table 7–2 Topical Flouride: Treatment Guidelines[a]

Age/Patient	No/Low Caries	Caries-Prone (2 or more/year)	Rampant Caries (several large lesions)
2 years and under	Fluoride dentrifice (small amount)	Fluoride dentrifice (small amount)	Fluoride dentrifice OTC rinse (1×/day)[b]—use for 1–2 months
2–6 years	Fluoride dentrifice (small amount)	Fluoride dentrifice OTC rinse (1×/day)[b] —use for 1–2 months	Fluoride dentrifice OTC rinse (1×/day)[b] or 0.4% SnF_2 gel (1×/day)[b]—use for 1–2 months
6 years and older	Fluoride dentrifice OTC rinse (1×/day) (optional)	Fluoride dentrifice OTC rinse (1×/day) or 0.05% NaF rinse (1×/day) or 0.044% APF rinse (1×/day) or 0.4% SnF_2 gel (1–2×/day) or 0.2% NaF rinse (1×/week)	Fluoride dentrifice OTC rinse (1×/day) or 0.05% NaF rinse (1×/day) or 0.044% APF rinse (1×/day) or 0.4% SnF_2 gel (1–2×/day) or 0.2% NaF rinse (1×/week) or 1.1% NaF gel (1×/day) or 1.1% APF gel (1×/day)—use until no caries
Patient wearing orthodontic appliances	Fluoride dentrifice OTC rinse (1×/day)	Fluoride dentrifice OTC rinse (1×/day) or 0.5 NaF rinse (1×/day) or 0.2% NaF rinse (1×/week) or 0.4% SnF_2 gel (1–2×/day) or 1.1% NaF gel (1×/day)	Fluoride dentrifice OTC rinse (1×/day) or 0.5 NaF rinse (1×/day) or 0.4% SnF_2 gel (1–2×/day) or 1.1% NaF gel (1×/day)

NaF: sodium fluoride; OTC: over-the-counter products; SnF_2: stannous fluoride; APF: acidulated phosphate fluoride.
[a]The above are suggested guidelines. The final decision for determining the proper fluoride supplements depends upon the professional's assessment of the patient's needs.
[b]These products are usually not recommended for children under the age of 6 years. Therefore, extreme caution should be taken. Apply these agents in very small amounts with either a cotton-tipped applicator or a small toothbrush.
Based on data from American Dental Association. (1994). *A guide to the use of fluorides for the prevention of dental caries.* Chicago, IL: Author. Wei, S.H.Y. (1985). *Clinical uses of fluorides.* Philadelphia: Lea & Febiger. Courtsey of M. Diane Melrose, RDH, BS.

Guided Practice Activities

(10 minutes)

This segment may be combined with the preceding instruction/information segment. Visual aids are included at the end of the lesson.

- Utilize small group discussions on various types and uses of fluorides (use the general information presented earlier to stimulate discussion).
- Review types of toothpastes, mouth rinses, and other products that contain fluoride. Display the fluoride ingredients on these product labels. Review the display of fluoride samples used in the anticipatory planning segment of this lesson.
- Identify the types of fluorides through the fluoride family album.
- Present the fluoride family play or story.
- Have the students draw a tooth that received fluoride (see handout).

FLUORIDE FAMILY ALBUM

Create your own album utilizing pictures of fluoride products. This lesson can be used as a lead-in to the fluoride family play, which follows.

Fluoride Family Story

The Fluoride Family Story

Read the following story to the class (grades K–2) or use as a play (grades 3–6) Pick eight students to represent Flo and the members of her family. The narrator can read the story, or the family members can read their own dialogue.

This is the story of Flo Fluoride and her family.

FAMILY MEMBERS:

Flo (narrator): fluoride drop
Freddy (father): fluoride gel
Florence (mother): fluoride in toothpaste
Fay (sister): fluoride rinse
Uncle Floyd: fluoride tablet
Frank and Frannie (cousins to Flo): fluoride in the water
Grandpa Fester: fluoride in foods

     Flo: My name is Flo Fluoride. You may not know who I am, but I know who you are. My family and I work day and night to keep your teeth healthy and strong. We are invisible while we go about our work, but today I have a special treat for you. You get to meet all of my family. Here I am! I'm hiding inside these fluoride drops that look like water. I'm a fluoride drop. I've helped your teeth since you were just a baby.

    Florence: Can you find me? I'm very busy at home. You can usually find me in your toothpaste. I help to protect your teeth every time you brush with a fluoride toothpaste. Do you have fluoride in your toothpaste?

    Freddy: I work at the dental clinic or office. I'm in the fluoride gel that the dentist or dental hygienist puts on your teeth. Fluoride gel protects your teeth with an invisible shield even after the gel is gone.

    Fay: I'm a fluoride rinse. Each time you swish the rinse around in your mouth, fluoride clings to your teeth to protect them. Can you name a fluoride rinse that you can find me in?

Uncle:	I'm a fluoride tablet. Every time you chew a fluoride tablet, I stand guard over
Floyd:	your teeth to make them strong.
Cousins Frannie and Frank:	We live at the water works, but we travel a lot. Sometimes we are added to the water before it goes through town and into your house or the drinking fountain at your school. Every time you drink water with fluoride, you are building stronger teeth. Be sure to drink water every day. Is there fluoride in your water?
Grandpa Fester:	I'm found in small amounts in the green leafy vegetables, fish, and tuna that you eat to make your bodies big and strong.
Flo:	I'm happy that you have been able to meet my family. I'm so proud of all the good work we do for you. The Fluoride family works every day to keep your teeth healthy and strong.

CLOSURE

(2–3 minutes)

- Restate the objectives in question form.
- Check students' knowledge and understanding of the concepts presented.
- If time permits, address any other questions the students may have. Relate the importance of fluoride to dental health.

Lesson Plan / FLUORIDE

Anticipatory Set

Bring samples of items that contain fluoride in a large basket (mouth rinse, toothpaste, floss, vitamins, water, green leafy vegetables, tea, etc.)
Question: Did you know that your teeth could last forever if we take care of them?

Objectives

Students will be able to distinguish between topical and systemic fluoride.
Student will be able to list two ways to get topical fluoride and 2 ways to get systemic fluoride
Students will be able to explain the benefits of fluoride

Instruction/Information

Visual: rock with fluoride (analogy that fluoride comes from rocks which are minerals) Discuss the items that contain fluoride, explain the difference between Systemic and Topical use flannel board discussion.
Methods: Students will break up into small groups to discuss the topical/systemic.

Guided Practice Activities

Hold up samples of items and ask if they agree it is topical or systemic use a thumbs up for agreement and thumbs down if disagreement. (toothpaste is systemic, thumbs down, should not be swallowed).

Closure

1. Name two examples of topical fluoride
2. Name two examples of systemic fluoride
3. Name one reason why fluoride is important (ask several times)
4. Explain what a topical fluoride is
5. Explain what a systemic fluoride is.

CHAPTER 8

Nutrition and Healthy Teeth

Nutrition as it relates to diet plays an important role in oral health and healthy teeth. The Dietary Guidelines for Americans 2005 booklet highlights the following on how you can "Feel better today, stay healthy for tomorrow." Eating right and getting plenty of physical activity will lead to a healthy lifestyle that may prevent and/or reduce your risk for certain cancers, heart disease, diabetes, osteoporosis, and many other chronic diseases. Make smart choices every day from each food group. The following are key recommendations from the Dietary Guidelines for Americans 2005*:

1. Make smart choices from every food group.
2. Find your balance between food and physical activity.
3. A wide range of calories have been set to accommodate the needs of different age groups, genders, and activity levels. See attached table Estimated Daily Calorie Needs.
   a. Children and adolescents are recommended to engage in at least an hour of physical activity each day.
4. Get the most nutrition out of your calories.
   a. Consume a variety of nutrient-dense foods and beverages within and among the basic food groups.
5. Mix up your choices within each food group.
   a. Focus on fruits and vegetables, whole-grain products, and fat-free or low-fat milk or equivalent milk products.
      i. Eat more dark green vegetables (dark leafy, broccoli), orange vegetables (carrots, sweet potatoes), starchy vegetables, and other vegetables (one cup of raw or cooked vegetables or vegetable juice; two cups of raw leafy greens count as one cup from the vegetable group).
      ii. Eat more fresh fruits rather than fruit juice (one cup of fruit, one small banana, one medium orange, or half cup of dried fruits).
      iii. Eat at least three ounces of whole grains per day (one slice bread, one cup ready-to-eat unsweetened cereal, or half cup cooked rice, pasta, or cooked cereal is considered as one ounce equivalent from the grain group).
   b. Get three cups of low-fat or fat-free milk or an equivalent amount of low-fat yogurt and/or low-fat cheese every day. For children aged 2–8 years, it is two cups of milk.
      i. In general, one cup of milk or yogurt, 1.5 ounces of natural cheese, or two ounces of processed cheese is considered as one cup from the milk group.
   c. Choose lean meats and poultry. Bake it, broil it, or grill it. Vary your protein choices with more fish, dry beans, peas, nuts, and seeds.
6. Read the Nutrition Facts label on packaged foods. The Nutrition Facts label can help you in making smart food choices.
   a. Look for foods low in saturated fats, *trans* fats, cholesterol, and sodium.
      i. Use the % Daily Value (% DV) column when making selections.
      ii. 5% DV or less is "low"; 10–19% DV is a "good source"; 20% DV or more is "high."

    b. Read the ingredient list to make sure that added sugar is not among the first three ingredients under the ingredient list.

       i. Names for added sugars include: sucrose, high fructose corn syrup, corn syrup, and fructose.

7. Water is also essential to keeping healthy. In fact, water is the most vital of all nutrients. Drink enough water to keep hydrated. Water is the nutrient that moves nutrients from foods throughout the body. Water helps to remove waste products from the body.

Source: Adapted from The Dietary Guidelines for Americans. U.S. Department of Health and Human Services. U.S. Department of Agriculture. www.healthierus .gov/dietaryguidelines

PREPARATION

(5 minutes before beginning lesson)

Assemble pictures or cards of foods; a picnic or a class party menu; a variety of packaged foods and snacks, some of which contain sugar, others of which are sugar-free; a chart of the food pyramid; and a 1-lb box of sugar. Bring information about nutrition from your local dairy council. Use Figure 8-1, Tables 8-1 and 8-2 for assistance.

ANTICIPATORY PLANNING

(5 minutes)

- Review the previous lesson, if applicable.
- Introduce presenters.
- Describe the goals of today's lesson, the format of information, and general topics to be covered.
- Review classroom rules (K–3), if applicable.
- Survey the class about current food choices. (Ask: What did you eat for breakfast?)
- Review the dental disease process (see Figure 4-1).

General Objectives by Grade Level

(2–3 minutes)

State specifically not more than three objectives appropriate for the classroom learning level that indicate what the majority of the students will be able to achieve by the completion of the lesson. Keep in mind that for every grade level you advance, the previous grade level objectives could also be used.

    Upon completion of this lesson, the student will be able to achieve the objectives listed in the following table.

GR	OBJECTIVE
K–1	State that a variety of foods are needed for health and to build strong bodies.
	Choose a variety of foods that are good for teeth.
	Identify the food groups and their place in the food pyramid.
2	State why foods are arranged in the pyramid the way that they are.
3	Include any or all of the above information.
4	Include any or all of the above information.
5	Include any or all of the above information.
6	Include any or all of the above information.

INSTRUCTION/INFORMATION

(10 minutes)

More than one topic may be included or combined with the guided practice segment (10–20 minutes). Use as many visuals as possible for grades K–3; group discussion may be more appropriate for grades 4–6.

- Explain why good nutrition is important.
- Present the food pyramid.
- Review the recommended daily requirements.
- Discuss the importance of dental nutrition.
- Relate the facts and myths of dental nutrition.

General Information

The food pyramid illustrates the principles of a healthy diet recommended by professionals and national health organizations. A balanced diet is important in preventing cavities; however, cavities are also the results of what we eat and how often these foods are eaten (Figure 8-1).

When we eat, particles of foods can become trapped on or between tooth surfaces. When refined carbohydrate foods such as bread, corn flakes, pasta, crackers, and potato chips are allowed to remain in the mouth without brushing, the bacteria that live in the mouth break down these starches into sugars. These sugars, in turn, are converted into acids that can eat away at tooth enamel. Frequent snacking leaves food on our teeth longer; thus, it is more apt to begin the decay process (see Figure 4-1). For this reason, sugars and starches are best reserved for mealtime when increased saliva production helps to neutralize the acid attack.

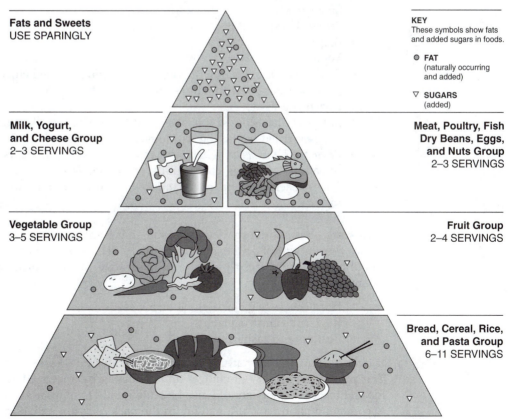

Fats and Sweets
USE SPARINGLY

KEY
These symbols show fats and added sugars in foods.

● **FAT**
(naturally occurring and added)

▽ **SUGARS**
(added)

Milk, Yogurt, and Cheese Group
2–3 SERVINGS

Meat, Poultry, Fish Dry Beans, Eggs, and Nuts Group
2–3 SERVINGS

Vegetable Group
3–5 SERVINGS

Fruit Group
2–4 SERVINGS

Bread, Cereal, Rice, and Pasta Group
6–11 SERVINGS

FIGURE 8–1 The Food Pyramid.

Acid-producing foods include:

- Cakes
- Candy
- Cookies
- Cough drops
- Doughnuts
- Gelatin dessert
- Gum
- Honey
- Jams
- Jellies
- Liqueurs
- Mints
- Molasses
- Pies
- Popsicles
- Soft drinks
- Syrup
- Table sugar

The texture of some foods causes them to be retained in the mouth longer than others. For instance, chocolates dissolve and clear the mouth quickly. However, raisins and sticky foods such as caramels, gumdrops, or peanut butter remain on the teeth for longer periods of time unless brushed off.

Some good snacks for children to eat are:

- Soft fruits
- Cooked vegetables
- Small sandwich
- String cheese
- Bagel
- Yogurt
- *Fast food choices*: Pizza with vegetable topping, broiled chicken sandwich, plain hamburger with lettuce and tomato, baked potato, milk, juice, and frozen yogurt.
- *Junk food choices:* Read the labels and eat healthy snacks such as popcorn, pretzels, dried fruits, yogurts, nuts, fruits, and fruit juice Popsicles.
- *Beware of TV advertising.* This can make you ask for many foods, like sweet cereals, potato chips, cheese puffs, candy, sodas, snack cakes, and cookies. These snacks are expensive and low in nutrition, high in fat, sugar, and salt.

Research has shown that certain foods have anticavity power, that is, they reduce the amount of acid exposure to the teeth. These foods are more dentally sound because they fight plaque and neutralize the acid-producing bacteria. Examples include:

- Hard cheese (e.g., Jack, cheddar, Swiss)
- Raw fruits and vegetables
- Peanuts and cashews

It is important to alternate these dentally preferred snacks in our daily diet. This provides a variety of choices and ensures a balanced intake of nutritious foods. Physical activity should also be added daily to maintain a healthy weight. Recommend taking a walk, playing in the park, playing ball, dancing to music, having a family playtime. Limit television to one to two hours per day.

The Food Pyramid

Each of the food groups in the food pyramid provides some, but not all, of the nutrients we need each day. Foods in one group cannot replace those in another group; therefore, no one food group is more important than any other. However, it is wise to limit solid fats, such as butter, stick margarine, shortening, and lard. These offer more calories than nutrients and may lead to unwanted weight gain. Choose foods and beverages low in added sugar for the same reason.

The number of servings from the different groups varies. These recommended daily servings ensure that we consume adequate nutrients while moderating the amount of fat, sugar, and calories in our diets (Tables 8-1 and 8-2).

This information can be modified for children in grades K–3 and 4–6 as noted below.

Grades K–3

The pyramid helps us to learn about the foods we need to have energy and healthy bodies. More of our servings should come from foods at the wider sections of the pyramid (vegetables, fruit, whole grains, and milk). However, it is still important to eat foods from all the food groups. As long as we are getting enough foods from the food groups to fill our pyramids it is okay to eat some "extras" in moderation or with our meals.

Table 8–1   Recommended Daily Requirements

	Number of Servings	
Food Group	*Age 5–9 years*	*Age 9 years–Adult*
Bread	6–9	6–11
Vegetables	3–4	3–5
Fruit	2–3	2–4
Milk	2–3	2–3
Meat	2–3	2–3
Extras (fats, oils, and sugars)		Use sparingly

Table 8–2   Hidden Dietary Sugar

Meal	Item (1 serving)	Sugar (tsp)
Breakfast	Fruit Loops cereal	4
	Doughnut	6
	Hot cocoa	6
	Tang	8
Lunch	Skippy peanut butter	1
	Jelly	3
	White bread (2 slices)	2.5
	Potato chips	1
	Pepsi	10
		48

Grades 4–6

The pyramid helps us to choose a variety of foods in proper amounts to keep our bodies healthy. Each food group gives us different essential nutrients, so it is important to eat foods from all the food groups everyday. When foods are eaten in the recommended amounts, we can be sure we will get our daily requirements for the nutrients we need to grow and feel great. More of our total servings should come from vegetables, fruit, whole grains, and milk, but that does not take the place of servings from the other groups. Eating "extras" is okay as long as they are not eaten instead of foods we need to fill up our pyramids. That is because these "extras" contain few if any nutrients. By following the recommended servings from each group, we also keep from getting too much fat and sugar.

Follow-up Activities: The Food Pyramid

- Have students plan a menu using food cards. See how many foods from the pyramid fit into three meals.
- Have students identify foods that would be good snacks.
- Have students tell what they brought for lunch. Have the class identify which foods fit into which groups in the pyramid.
- Review the foods and serving sizes required for each group by building the "Great Food Pyramid."
- Ask students to keep track of the foods they eat for one week. In the next lesson, ask whether they met the daily requirements of the food pyramid.

Dental Nutrition

Although sugar is an essential part of the diet, refined sugar consumption among Americans has skyrocketed out of control. Because sugar has a primary role in dental diseases, it should be apparent that nutrition education is a vital part of dental education.

Healthy teeth are possible for most people if knowledge of dental disease is used to alter unhealthy habits. Refined sugar is difficult to eliminate totally from the diet, but the form, frequency, and timing of sugar consumption can be altered. By improving nutritional knowledge and fostering a change in habits, we can help assure better dental health for most people.

Discussion: Facts and Myths of Dental Nutrition

Present the following facts:

- The average American will consume approximately his or her own weight in sugar in one year.
- The longer sugar stays in the mouth and the more frequently sweets are eaten, the more opportunity acids have to form.
- Sweets are less harmful to the teeth if eaten with a main meal rather than between meals.
- Liquid sweets are somewhat less harmful than sticky sweets.
- Table sugar is more harmful than sugars that occur naturally in fruits and milk.

Debunk the following myths:

- Eating apples, celery, and carrots *does not* aid significantly in plaque removal.
- Brushing your teeth or rinsing your mouth immediately after eating sweets is *not* an effective means of inhibiting acid formation.

- Natural sugars such as honey, molasses, corn sweetener, and raw sugar have the same acid-producing effects as refined sugar.

Note: All of the above statements are false.

Xylitol

Xylitol is a natural sweetener that can be found in fruits such as strawberries. This natural sugar alcohol helps to prevent cavities. It is contained in many sugarless products (gums and mints) that have mannitol and sorbitol. This particular sweetener shows the greatest promise for reducing tooth decay. Xylitol inhibits the bacteria (streptococcus mutants) that are known to cause cavities. Gum or mints with xylitol used three to five times daily, with a total intake of 5 grams is considered optimal. Xylitol has been shown effective in preventing tooth decay especially when combined with healthy eating habits for those people at moderate to high risk for decay.

Guided Practice Activities

(10 minutes)   This segment may be combined with the instruction/information segment. Visual aids are included at the end of the lesson.

- Perform the hidden sugar demonstration.
- Demonstrate how students can read the labels of various food products to identify those containing sugar.
- Have students find the super snack words in the puzzle (see handout).
- Relate the story of Happy Tooth and Sad Tooth.
- Have the students draw Happy Tooth and Sad Tooth (see handout).

HIDDEN SUGAR DEMONSTRATION

First, relate the average sugar intake per adult per year in the United States (about 135 lbs). Show a 1 lb or 5 lb box of sugar to illustrate. Next, state the amount of refined sugar our bodies require (zero). Emphasize that we get all the sugar we need from the sugar found naturally in fruits and vegetables. Explain the role of sugar in tooth decay (see Figure 4-1).

The following activity helps to illustrate how we manage to consume so much sugar, often without realizing it, during our daily meals and snacks. Describe a hypothetical breakfast, lunch, and afternoon snack of a school student. Write the menu items on the black/white board. Place a teaspoonful of table sugar into a clear glass, spoonful by spoonful, to indicate the amount of sugar in each item of the sample menu. Have students calculate the amount of sugar in each food item. (*Note*: 1 teaspoon = 3 grams.)

READING THE LABELS

The following activities can help to increase students' awareness of the sugar found in the food they eat each day:

1. Using the food label guide (provided at the end of this chapter) discuss the parts of Labels 1–6. Starting with the serving size through the footnote section.
2. Explain that all packaged foods are required by law to list ingredients, serving size, calories, calories from fat, the nutrients and how much, the

percentage of daily value based on a 2,000 calorie diet, and the upper limit and lower limit of the daily value. The older the population of participants is, the more time you can spend on reading labels.

3. Assemble a variety of packaged foods and snacks, some of which contain sugar, others of which are sugar-free. Enlarge the label and ingredients section to poster size. Explain that the ingredients are always displayed in order of their amount by weight in the product. Ask participants to explain what a "junk food" is. (*Answer*: Junk food is defined as a food that contains more sugar than nutrients.) Tell participants that junk foods can be identified by looking at food product labels. Junk foods are those foods that list sugar or a word meaning sugar as the first or second ingredient.

4. Show a poster of or list on the blackboard various words that indicate sugar: syrup, honey, molasses, sweeteners, and any word ending in "-ose."

5. Ask participants how we can determine whether a food has sugar in it. (*Answer*: Read labels, read recipes, and taste for sweetness.)

6. Have students (K–6) find the super snack words (words without sugar) in the word puzzle (see handout). Encourage students (K–12) to choose a sugar-free snack after school, at least for the day. Ask participants to promise to read the ingredients on the next packaged product they eat.

7. A child-friendly version of MyPyramid for teachers and children is being developed. Visit their website at www.heathierus.gov/dietaryguidelines.

Happy Tooth and Sad Tooth

Happy Tooth and Sad Tooth

Assemble the following supplies:

Two pieces of 18 × 24-inch easel paper, to be taped to the blackboard or pinned to the wall
Markers in two colors
Pictures of food cut out of magazines and newspaper ads

Today's story is about two molar teeth. Do any of you know which teeth are molars? They are the teeth way in the back of your mouth. Put your tongue on your very back tooth. Feel what a big tooth it is? Some of you have brand new molars there. These are permanent teeth that will not fall out. They are supposed to last forever, so we must take good care of them.

The first story is about a happy, healthy molar. This tooth uses fluoride to be strong, it brushes to get rid of plaque, it flosses to keep the sides clean and healthy, and it visits the dentist regularly. This tooth eats good foods like fruits, vegetables, and cheese. (Have the class suggest some other good foods.) It looks good and feels good because it takes good care of itself. This tooth will be easy to draw because we all know it. Do you know its name? (*Happy Tooth.*)

Now I am going to tell you about another molar. This tooth forgets to brush, floss, or use fluoride. It does not feel well and it does not look well. What is its name? (*Sad Tooth.*) Can you imagine what kinds of food Sad Tooth eats? (Have students name a few.)

Follow-up Activities: Happy Tooth and Sad Tooth

1. Have the students draw Happy Tooth and Sad Tooth using the following script:
   a. Draw Happy Tooth first. Start with the crown. (Describe what the crown is.) Next, draw the roots, which are the feet and legs of a tooth. (Explain that the roots hold the teeth in our mouths. Permanent teeth have long roots, and molars have two or three roots.) Put the happy eyes, nose, smiling mouth, strong arms, and smooth cape on Happy Tooth. Happy Tooth takes good care of itself and eats nutritious foods.

b. Now let us draw Sad Tooth. Is it healthy? Is it happy? How will we begin? What does Sad Tooth's crown look like? Draw a molar with holes in the top. Have the students complete the drawing as for Happy Tooth, adding weak arms, short roots, sad face, torn cape, etc.

2. Place the pictures of food you have cut out of magazines and newspaper ads in a lunch bag. Half of the pictures should be of healthful foods, the other half of not healthful foods. Ask the class to indicate which are good food choices and which are bad food choices. Tape the pictures around the appropriate tooth picture. Leave the pictures in the classroom to help remind students to make good food choices. Tell them to bring in pictures to add around the appropriate tooth. Emphasize how Sad Tooth could become happy.

CLOSURE

(2–3 minutes)

- Restate the objectives in question form.
- Check students' knowledge and understanding of the concepts presented.
- If time permits, address any other questions the students may have.

READING LABELS (FIGURE 8-2)

No. 1: Serving Size

Serving sizes are standardized to make it easier to compare similar foods. Pay attention to the serving size, especially how many servings there are in the food package.

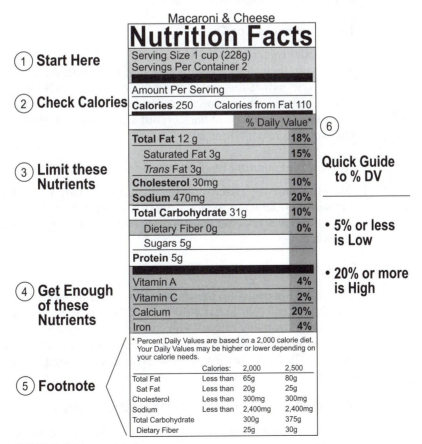

FIGURE 8–2 Nutrition Label.

Then ask yourself how many servings are you consuming. In the sample label, one serving of macaroni and cheese equals one cup. If you eat the whole package, you would eat two cups. That doubles the calories and other nutrient numbers, including the % Daily Values as shown in the sample label.

No. 2: Calories (and Calories from Fat)

Calories provide a measure of how much energy you get from a serving of this food. Remember: the number of servings you consume determines the number of calories you actually eat. In the sample, there are 250 calories in one serving of this macaroni and cheese. How many calories from fat are there in one serving? Answer: 110, which means almost half of the calories in a single serving come from fat. What if you ate the whole package content? Then you would consume two servings, or 500 calories, and 220 would come from fat.

> General Guide to Calories Based on 2,000 Calorie Diet: 40 calories is low, 100 calories is moderate, and 400 calories is high. Eating too many calories per day is linked to overweight and obesity.

Nos. 3 and 4: The Nutrients: How Much?

Separate the nutrients into two main groups.

No. 3: Limit These Nutrients

The nutrients listed first are the ones Americans generally eat in adequate amounts, or even too much. Saturated fat, *trans* fat, cholesterol, and sodium. Health experts recommend that you keep your intake of these as low as possible as part of a nutritionally balanced diet.

No. 4: Get Enough of These

Most Americans do not get enough dietary fiber, vitamin A, vitamin C, calcium, and iron in their diets. Eating enough of these nutrients can improve your health and help to reduce the risk of some diseases and conditions.

Remember, you can use the Nutrition Facts label not only to help limit those nutrients you want to cut back on but also to increase those nutrients you need to consume in greater amounts.

No. 5: Understanding the Footnote on the Bottom of the Nutrition Facts Label

Note the asterisk (*) used after the heading "% Daily Value (DV)" on the Nutrition Facts label. It refers to the footnote in the lower part of the nutrition label, which tells you that % DVs are based on a 2,000 calorie diet. This statement must be on all food labels.

No. 6: The Percent Daily Value (% DV)

The % DV are based on the Daily Value recommendations for key nutrients, but only for a 2,000 calorie daily diet—not 2,500 calories. Like most people, you may not know how many calories you consume in a day. However, you can still use the % DV as a frame of reference whether or not you consume more or less than 2,000 calories. The % DV helps you to determine if a serving of food is high or low in a nutrient.

5% DV or Less Is Low and 20% DV or More Is High

Example: Look at the amount of total fat in one serving listed on the sample nutrition label. Is 18% DV contributing a lot or a little to your fat limit of 100% DV? The

18% for one serving is not that high, but if you eat the whole package you would consume 36% DV of total fat allowance, which is considered high.

Nutrients with a % DV but No Weight Listed

Calcium: Look at the % DV for calcium on food packages so you know how much one serving contributes to the total amount you need per day. Remember a food with 20% DV or more contributes a lot of calcium to your daily total, while one with 5% DV or less contributes a little. Experts advise adult consumers to consume adequate amounts of calcium, that is, 1,000 mg or 100% DV in a daily 2,000-calorie diet.

Visit the website: www.MyPyramid.gov for the latest details and updates of the USDA's information. MyPyramid is intended to reach children 6–11 years old with targeted messages about the importance of making smart choices in eating and physical activities. The Dietary Guidelines for Americans 2005 and consumer brochure are available at www.healthierus.gov/dietaryguidelines (Table 8-3).

Table 8–3 Healthy Foods Word Search

Name_____

Find the supersnack words (words without sugar) in this puzzle. (Hint: Words may be found across, backward, down, or diagonally.)

M	C	E	L	E	R	Y	P	Z	S
B	I	T	H	E	E	T	E	G	G
U	P	L	Y	S	O	Z	A	M	T
Z	V	R	K	G	O	N	N	R	P
A	P	P	L	E	R	P	U	H	E
A	T	A	I	O	U	J	T	C	G
R	A	F	C	H	E	E	S	E	N
D	C	P	V	K	D	H	B	P	A
S	O	C	A	R	R	O	T	Q	R
P	W	J	A	Z	Z	I	P	M	O

Can you find the following words?

Apple	Carrot	Cheese	Taco
Celery	Popcorn	Egg	Peanuts
Milk	Orange	Pizza	

Name_____

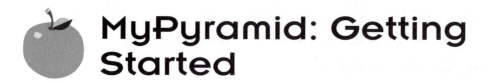

MyPyramid: Getting Started

USDA has released the MyPyramid food guidance system (www.mypyramid.gov). Along with the new MyPyramid symbol, the system provides many options to help Americans make healthy food choices and to be active every day. Below is information that can help you navigate through the new MyPyramid system to educate consumers.

MyPyramid symbol—*Explain the message in the MyPyramid symbol.* These are physical activity, variety, proportionality, moderation, gradual improvement, and finally personalization. More information on these messages can be found on the "Anatomy of MyPyramid" handout.

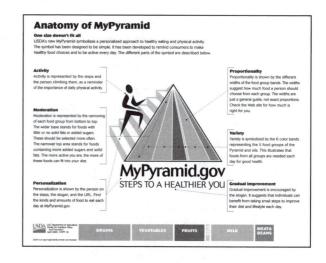

MyPyramid's Basic Messages—*Give consumers MyPyramid's basic messages about healthy eating and physical activity, which apply to everyone.* These can be found on the miniposter and the website. They mirror the messages from the 2005 Dietary Guidelines for Americans consumer brochure. For example:

- Eat at least 3 ounces of whole-grain cereals, rice, or pasta every day;
- Go low-fat or fat-free when you choose milk, yogurt, and other milk products and
- Choose food and beverages low in added sugars.

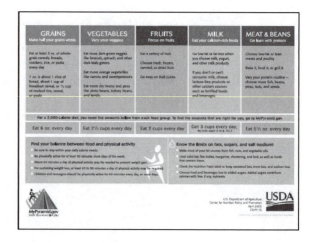

MyPyramid Plan—*Help consumers find the kinds and amounts of foods they should ear each day at MyPyramid.gov.* When they enter their age, gender, and activity level, they get their own plan at an appropriate calorie level. The food plan includes specific daily amounts from each food group and a limit for discretionary calories (fats, added sugars, alcohol). Their food plan is one of the 12 calorie levels of the food intake patterns from the Dietary Guidelines. They can print out a personalized miniposter of their plan, and a worksheet to help them track their progress and choose goals for tomorrow and the future.

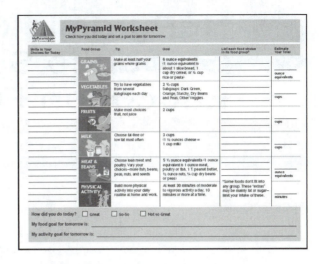

Inside the Pyramid—*Point consumers to the in-depth information about each food group, discretionary calories, and physical activity on the website at "Inside the Pyramid."* Here they can find tips and resources to help them implement their food plan. For example:

- what counts as an ounce of grain?
- what foods are in each group?
- tips for incresing whole grain consumption and limiting solid fats
- food photo gallery to help identify portion sizes
- and many more. . . .

Additional information can be found at "Tips and Resources" and "For Professionals", such as a 7-day menu plan at 2000 calories and tips for eating out. www.mypramid.gov/tips_resources/index.html www.mypyramid.gov/professionals/index.html

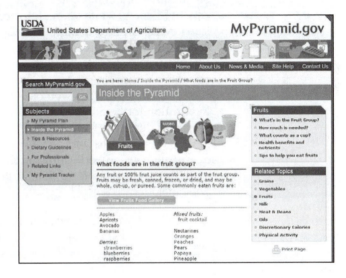

MyPyramid Tracker—*For consumers who want a detailed assessment and analysis of their current eating and physical activity habits, have them try MyPyramid Tracker* (www.mypyramidtracker.gov/). This dietary and physical activity assessment tool asks for entry of all foods eaten each day and all physical activities performed. Form this, a wealth of output shows their current status in comparison to the 2005 Dietary Guidelines recommendations, nutrient intake, and energy balance. A history function allows consumers to track their progress over time, up to one year.

The 2005 Dietary Guidelines (DG) Recommendations for JohnDoe on 4/11/2005

Click directly on the 😊😐☹️ emoticon (face) for more detailed dietary information.

Dietary Guidelines Recommendations	Emoticon	Number of cup/ oz. Equ. Eaten	Number of cup/oz. Equ. Recommended
Grain	😊	5.7 oz equivalent	6 oz equivalent
Vegetable	😊	2 cup equivalent	2.5 cup equivalent
Fruit	☹️	0.8 cup equivalent	2 cup equivalent
Milk	😐	2 cup equivalent	3 cup equivalent
Meat and Beans	😊	5.2 oz equivalent	5.5 oz equivalent

Dietary Guidelines Recommendations	Emoticon	Amount Eaten	Recommendation or Goal
Total Fat	☹️	45.9% of total calories	20% to 35%
Saturated Fat	☹️	14.6% of total calories	less than 10%
Cholesterol	😊	258 mg	less than 300 mg
Sodium	☹️	7406 mg	less than 2300 mg
Oils	*	*	*
Discretionary calories (solid fats, added sugars, and alcohol)	*	*	*

Source: Center for Nutrition Policy and Promotion April 2005

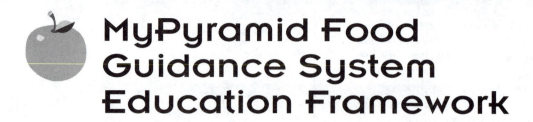

MyPyramid Food Guidance System Education Framework

BACKGROUND

The 2005 Dietary Guidelines for Americans are the basis for Federal nutrition policy. The MyPyramid Food Guidance System provides food-based guidance to help implement the recommendations of the Guidelines. MyPyramid was based on both the Guidelines and the Dietary Reference Intakes from the National Academy of Sciences, while taking into account current consumption patterns of Americans. MyPyramid translates the Guidelines into a *total diet* that meets nutrient needs from food sources and aims to moderate or limit dietary components often consumed in excess. An important complementary tool is the Nutrition Facts label on food products.

MyPyramid provides web-based interactive and print materials for consumers. In addition to the materials developed for consumers, MyPyramid also includes materials designed for professionals. These professional materials are intended for use by programs and agencies in developing consumer education materials; by nutritionists and educators as the basis for their education efforts; and by the media to assist them in understanding and reporting of Federal food guidance. They include:

- *Food Intake Patterns* that identify *what* and *how much* food an individual should eat for health. The amounts to eat are based on a person's age, sex, and activity level. These patterns have been published in the 2005 Dietary Guidelines.
- *Education Framework* that explains *what changes* most Americans need to make in their eating and activity choices, *how* they can make these changes, and *why* these changes are important for health.
- *Glossary* that defines key terms used in the MyPyramid Food Guidance System documents.

This document includes the Education Framework and the Glossary.

OVERVIEW OF MYPYRAMID FOOD GUIDANCE SYSTEM EDUCATION FRAMEWORK

The MyPyramid Education Framework provides specific recommendations for making food choices that will improve the quality of an average American diet. These recommendations are interrelated and should be used together. Taken together, they would result in the following changes from a typical diet:

- Increased intake of vitamins, minerals, dietary fiber, and other essential nutrients, especially of those that are often low in typical diets.
- Lowered intake of saturated fats, *trans* fats, and cholesterol and increased intake of fruits, vegetables, and whole grains to decrease risk for some chronic diseases.

- Calorie intake balanced with energy needs to prevent weight gain and/or promote a healthy weight.

The recommendations in this Education Framework fall under four overarching themes:

- **Variety**—Eat foods from all food groups and subgroups.
- **Proportionality**—Eat more of some foods (fruits, vegetables, whole grains, fat-free or low-fat milk products), and less of others (foods high in saturated or *trans* fats, added sugars, cholesterol salt, and alcohol).
- **Moderation**—Choose forms of foods that limit intake of saturated or *trans* fats, added sugars, cholesterol, salt, and alcohol.
- **Activity**—Be physically active every day.

The Framework's recommendations are presented as key concepts for educators. The key concepts are organized by topic area: calories; physical activity; grains; vegetables; fruits; milk, yogurt, and cheese; meat, poultry, fish, dry beans, eggs, and nuts; fats and oils; sugars and sweets; salt; alcohol; and food safety. Under each topic area, information is presented on:

- *What* actions should be taken for a healthy diet,
- *How* these actions can be implemented, and
- *Why* this action is important for health (the key benefits).

These key concepts are not intended as direct consumer messages, but rather as a framework of ideas from which professionals can develop consumer messages and materials.

* Visit website www.mypyramid.gov/professionals for additional and current information.

Lesson Plan / NUTRITION

Anticipatory Set

Create awareness of healthy eating habits; good food vs bad foods, and super tooth helps to make good choices.
Posters or food cards with pictures of good and bad foods.

Objectives

1. State and or relate that a variety of foods help them grow.

2. State and or relate that you need to make smart choices from every food group.

3. State and or relate why daily physical activity is also important.

Instruction

Visit www.mypyramid.gov for undated information on food choices, use information available for charts, pictures etc.
Review the pyramid appropriate for the grade level presenting to.
Review the importance of daily physical activities for good health.
Review the importance of healthy teeth and making food choices.

Guided Practice Activities

Sugar demo
Discuss food facts and read labels
Food pyramid

Closure

Restate objectives in question form
Check for individual knowledge
Independent practice
Word search puzzle

CHAPTER 9

Dental Sealants

INFORMATION

SEALANTS ARE USED TO PROTECT CHILDREN'S TEETH FROM CAVITIES

Healthy People 2010 calls for half of all U.S. children to have dental sealants by 2010. Currently fewer than 25 percent of school-age children do. Sealants are a plastic coating (resin) applied to the chewing surfaces of the back teeth. They are a safe and effective way to aid in preventing cavities among school children. The sealant provides a physical barrier (shield) to prevent cavity-causing bacteria from invading the pits and fissures on a tooth. Sealants can be chemical or light cure. They are easy to apply to the tooth surface and only take a few minutes for each tooth. The sealant is most effective in newly formed teeth after complete eruption (age 6–12 years old). Many school districts, county health programs, and all private practices are providing sealants for school-age children as part of an integrated dental disease prevention program. Sealants may last from 5 to 10 years.

Sealants should not be used as an alternative to fluorides (toothpaste, varnishes, mouth rinses, etc.). Fluorides work best on the smooth surfaces and not on the chewing surfaces of the back teeth. Sealants and fluorides work together to prevent tooth decay.

Mary and Mikey Molar

Mary and Mikey Molar Get Sealants

Create your own visuals to accompany this story, describing the procedure for applying a sealant.

Mary and Mikey are two molars that have just erupted. The tops (chewing surface) of Mary and Mikey Molar are very groovy. The two molars are worried about getting germs that can turn into decay. (Check students' knowledge of the meaning of the word "decay.") Mary and Mikey visit the dentist, who tells them that the dentist or the dental hygienist can put a special coating on the grooves that will prevent germs (seal out the decay) from getting into the tooth. Mary and Mikey think this is a good idea.

First Mary sits down in the dental chair. She sees the hose for water and for air. Mary's top enamel is brushed and cleaned with a small electric brushing machine. Next comes a liquid that has a bitter taste (like lemons). With a dab of cotton, the liquid is put around the molar. After a minute, there is a water spray. Mary needs to be very dry before the sealant can be applied. Once the sealant has been applied, a bright light may be placed over the tooth to help it dry. When the procedure is over, the top of Mary's tooth feels nice and smooth. Then it is Mikey's turn to get his sealant.

When Mary and Mikey leave the dentist's office, they are happy. They know that now they have sealants that will protect their tops (chewing surface).

Suzie Sealant

Suzie Sealant

This is a story about the job of my friend Suzie Sealant.

"My name is Suzie Sealant. Some of you may have already met me." (Pause. Ask by show of hands if anyone has a sealant.)

"While many of you may not know who I am, I know who all of you are. I work hard to protect your teeth and keep them healthy by not allowing the plaque to attack and make cavities. Do you know what a cavity is?" (Pause for the participants to respond.)

"My job works best when I am placed on your teeth at a young age. You find me on your back teeth, along the biting surface." (Using a tooth model, show the biting or top surface where the sealant would be placed.)

"I am clear or white. Sometimes you cannot see me on your tooth but you can feel that I am there." (Explain the similarities to clear nail polish, and the smoothness on your nails.) "Today I am going to show you what I do at work."

"Your back teeth have tiny grooves. Sometimes its hard to brush way back there and remove the sticky plaque and germs that get into those grooves and cause cavities."

Create a picture of Suzie Sealant covering teeth using Figure 9-1 (Suzie Sealant). "Here I am doing my work in the back of your teeth."

Use Figure 5-2 (tooth and brush). "First, the tooth must be cleaned and free of any germs. The dental professional can clean the tooth surface with a brush."

Draw the liquid gel dropping onto the teeth using Figure 9-1A.

"Next a liquid gel called *etch* is placed on the tooth and then washed off. At this time the tooth must be very dry so that I will stay on the tooth surface."

Hold up Figure 9-1B. "Finally, I am painted on your tooth. It take about one minute to turn into a protective shield. Sometimes a magic bright light will be used to help me with this process. I keep the germs out of the grooves in your tooth, because now your tooth has a protective shield called a sealant."

"Now I am happy because you know how to protect your teeth. Since my work is only on the back teeth, I cannot be seen when you talk or smile (Figure 9-1C). But you know that I am there doing my job!"

Remember what Suzie Sealant says:

"Sealants are groovy because they save grooves!"

Follow-up questions and discussion

1. Identify areas where participants could go to get a sealant *(DDS office, public health, or school site if providing)*.
2. Name the type of teeth that sealants would be placed on.
3. Describe the procedures for placing a sealant.
4. Describe the purpose of placing a sealant.
5. Describe the benefit of sealants.

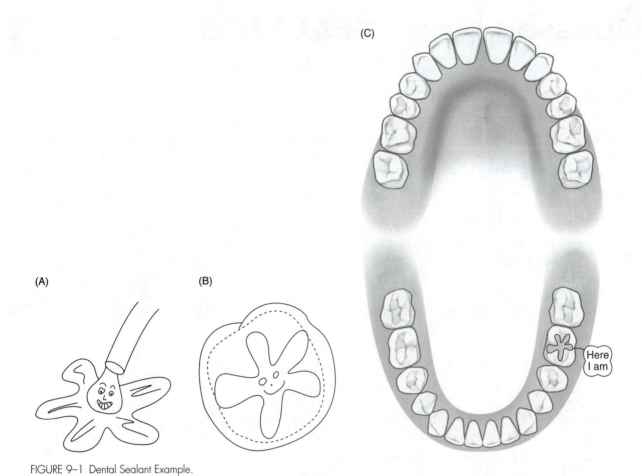

(A)   (B)   (C)

Here I am

FIGURE 9–1 Dental Sealant Example.

Lesson Plan / SEALANTS

Preparation

(5 minutes before beginning the lesson)

Assemble the necessary supplies, have samples of teeth with sealants (extracted teeth mounted in plaster, seal occlusal surfaces, typodont teeth with sealants applied). Tray set with samples of sealant materials, etching gel, mirror, explorer, etc.

Anticipatory Planning

- Review the previous lesson
- Introduce presenters
- Ask for volunteers (if applicable)
- Describe the goals of today's lesson
- Review classroom rules (if applicable)

General Objectives

Upon completion of this lesson, the student should be able to:

1. Describe what a sealant is.
2. Describe the benefit of a sealant.
3. Describe which teeth sealants are placed on.
4. Relate the procedure for placing a sealant.
5. Identify places where participants could go to get sealants.

Instructions/Information

Discuss how sealants are used to protect children's teeth from cavities.

Sealants can be placed directly on the tooth surface and will protect the tooth by sealing up the grooves that can easily become carious. Sealants can be chemical or light cure. They are easy to apply to the tooth surface and will take a few minutes for each tooth. The sealant is most effective in newly formed teeth after complete eruption. Many school districts, county health programs, and all private practices are providing sealants for school age children as part of an integrated dental disease prevention program. Sealants may last from 5–10 years.

Activities

Mary and Mikey Molar Sealants.
Suzie Sealant Story.
Diagrams 1–8 can be enlarged and placed on tongue blades to be shown or posted on a board, or used volunteers to hold up the pictures.
Sealant Fact Sheet information (appendix section).

CHAPTER 10

Dental Safety and Oral Injury Prevention

PREPARATION

(5 minutes before beginning lesson)

Display an easy-to-make dental emergency kit; dental emergency procedures wall chart, protective equipment (mouth guard, face protector, etc.), and safety signs.

ANTICIPATORY PLANNING

(5 minutes)

- Review the previous lesson, if applicable.
- Introduce presenters.
- Describe the goals of today's lesson, the format of information, and general topics to be covered.
- Review classroom rules (K–3), if applicable.
- Survey the class about how many students wear protective gear when playing sports. (Ask: Why is safety important to our teeth?)

General Objectives by Grade Level

(2–3 minutes)

State specifically not more than three objectives appropriate for the classroom learning level that indicate what the majority of the students will be able to achieve by the completion of the lesson. Keep in mind that for every grade level you advance, the previous grade level objectives could also be used.

Upon completion of this lesson, the student will be able to achieve the objectives listed in the following table.

GR	Objective
K	Name the dental safety rules.
1	Explain what do if a tooth is accidentally knocked out.
2	Explain the contents and purpose of a dental emergency kit.
3	Describe what to do for various dental emergencies.
4	Explain the importance of wearing protective mouth guards for various sports activities.
5	Describe the various types of mouth guards and why they are used for protection and safety.
6	Include any or all of the above information.

INSTRUCTION/INFORMATION

(15–20 minutes)

More than one topic may be included or combined with the guided practice segment (10–20 minutes). Use as many visuals as possible for grades K–3; group discussion may be more appropriate for grades 4–6.

- Present the dental safety rules.
- Describe the contents of a dental emergency kit.
- Discuss first aid for dental emergencies.
- Explain the different types of protective equipment that should be worn for various sports and play activities.
- Describe food safety rules and ways to prevent choking.

Dental Safety Rules

Use discussion, visual aids such as posters, or a guided practice activity to teach the following safety rules. Emphasize that many injuries that involve the teeth are preventable. By following good safety rules, you can prevent these types of injuries to your teeth.

Twelve Rules for Dental Safety

1. *Water/puddles:*   Always walk, do not run, around pools; be careful when walking on rainy days.

2. *Fighting:*   This is not the way to solve problems. It is better to walk away, ask for help, or talk it out with the person.

3. *Stairs:*   Walk, do not run, up and down stairs. Hold onto the banister. Do not slide down the banister.

4. *Seat-belts:*   Keep belts fastened at all times when riding in a car.

5. *Chewing on things:*   Hard objects such as ice can fracture a tooth. Sucking on lemons can also damage the teeth.

6. *Baseball games:*   Do not swing or throw the bat when someone is standing near you. Always wear a helmet. Put the glove in front of your face when catching the ball.

7. *Swing sets* : Do not stand or jump on or off the swing. Be careful of others standing close to your swing.

8. *Reaching for things in high places:*   Do not stand on a chair with wheels. Ask an adult for help.

9. *Ladder:* Check the equipment before climbing on it. Be sure a parent is nearby.

10. *Rocks:* Watch where you are walking. It is easy to trip over rocks or other objects when you are not looking in front of you.

11. *Drinking fountain:*   Do not push or shove or fool around in line while at the drinking fountain.

12. *Objects that do not belong in your mouth:*   Object such as pencils, paper clips, and coins can break or chip your teeth. The only things you should put in your mouth are food, toothbrushes, and floss.

13. *Food safety:* Avoid choking, cut food into small bite size pieces and do not talk while chewing.

Dental Emergency Kit

Every home and classroom should have a dental emergency kit available so that proper dental first aid can be administered when injuries occur. Many schools already have some of these items as part of their general first-aid kit. Be sure to provide the name(s) of a local dentist who can be contacted in case of an emergency if a family does not have one. Use Figure 10-1 for an in-class worksheet.

The kit should contain the following supplies:

- Cotton and cotton swabs to clean the injury.
- Dental floss, interdental cleaner, and toothpicks to remove objects from between the teeth.
- Dental wax or candle to stop irritation to cheeks or gums from a chipped tooth or orthodontic wires.
- Handkerchief, tie, or towel to immobilize a broken jaw.
- Ice pack to help reduce swelling.
- Medications (consult the school nurse or health aide).
- Hank's solution, Save-a-Tooth, cold milk, sterile gauze, or a clean cloth to provide temporary storage for a knocked-out tooth.

Dental Emergency Procedures

Teachers and students should know how to provide first aid for the most common dental emergencies. Present information on simple first-aid techniques for the following dental problems and emergencies.

Bitten Tongue

Apply direct pressure to the site of the irritation, and cover the bleeding area with a sterile or clean cloth. If swelling is present, apply cold compresses. If the bleeding does not stop readily or the bite is severe, take the child to the hospital emergency department.

Broken Tooth

Try to clean dirt or debris from the injured area with warm water. Place a cold compress on the face next to the injured tooth to minimize swelling. Take the child to the dentist immediately.

Knocked-out Tooth

Place the tooth in water, Hank's solution, or a Save-a-Tooth container, or wrap it in a clean, wet cloth. *Do not clean the tooth!* Take the child and the tooth to the dentist immediately.

Objects Wedged between the Teeth

Try to remove the object with dental floss. Guide the floss in carefully so as not to cut the gums. If unsuccessful, take the child to a dentist. *Do not* try to remove wedged objects using a sharp or pointed object.

Orthodontia Problems

Take the child to the orthodontist if:

- A wire is causing irritation.
- A wire is embedded in the cheek, tongue, or gum tissue.

Do not attempt to remove loose or broken appliances.

Possible Fractured Jaw

If a fracture is suspected, immobilize the jaw by any means (handkerchief, towel) and take the child to the hospital emergency department immediately.

Toothache

Rinse the mouth vigorously with warm water to clean out debris. Use dental floss to remove any food that might be trapped within the cavity. If swelling is present, apply cold compresses to the outside of the cheek. (Do not use heat.) *Do not* place aspirin on the gum tissue or aching tooth. Take the child to the dentist.

Food Safety

- Wash your hands with soap and water before eating or touching your food.
- Wash fresh vegetables and fruits before eating.
- Avoid burning your mouth by letting hot food cool down before eating.
- Sit down while eating.
- Do not give nuts, hard candy, popcorn, or raw vegetables to children under the age of 3 years.
- Do not run or play with food in your mouth.
- Do not get distracted while eating, which may lead to choking on food particles.
- Cut foods into small, manageable pieces to eat: hot dogs lengthwise into quarters, grapes in halves.
- Cook vegetables until tender.
- Learn the Heimlich maneuver to aid someone who might be choking.

Protective Equipment

Use Table 10-1 for assistance. Emphasize that protective equipment should be worn for all sports and play activities that can result in dental or other injuries. A mouth guard is a flexible piece of plastic that fits into the mouth. This device should be worn during all recreational and athletic activities (football, soccer, wrestling, baseball, lacrosse, hockey, martial arts, boxing, etc.) to protect the teeth from serious injury, especially during contact sports. Many other recreational activities (skateboarding, bicycling, etc.) pose a risk for mouth and teeth injury. Students should also be aware of simple safety measures that can prevent injuries during these activities. Injuries to the teeth, mouth, and head may include:

- Concussion
- Fractured jaw or neck injury
- Bitten or lacerated tongue and or lip
- Knocked-out tooth or teeth
- Broken or chipped tooth
- Objects caught between the teeth

Table 10–1   Protective Equipment and Safety Tips for Sports/Play Activities

Sport/Play Activity	Prevention
Football	Wear mouth guard, helmet
Baseball	Wear catcher's mask, helmet
Basketball	Wear mouth guard
Running games	Never trip; watch out for dangerous objects
Swimming and diving	Do not push; do not run; use a ladder
Tree climbing	Watch footing
Bicycling	Wear helmet; use care on wet roads and dirt
Skateboarding	Wear mouth guard, helmet, wrist, and knee bands
Roller skating	Control speed; wear helmet, wrist, and knee bands
Playground	Do not push or trip
Hill climbing	Check for firm footing
Soccer	Wear mouth guard, shin guards

*Source: Adapted with permission from *Prevention of Oral Injuries* Flip Chart, sponsored by the Dental Health Foundation and California Department of Health Services, Dental Health Section, Sacramento, CA; courtesy of Andrea Azevedo.

**Source: Courtesy of Kate Varanelli, RDH, MS, Sacramento SBIII.

Guided Practice Activities

(10 minutes)

This segment may be combined with the preceding instruction/information segment. Visual aids are included at the end of the lesson.

- Make a dental emergency kit for the classroom. Have students list the items to be included in the kit (see handout).
- Have students review the Play Safe worksheet (Figure 10-2). Students in grades K–3 can color in the pictures of each safety problem. Ask the students to explain what the teeth are doing wrong in each picture.
- Have students list the safety rules (see handout).
- Have students dress up in protective equipment.

CLOSURE

(2–3 minutes)

- Restate the objectives in question form.
- Check students' knowledge and understanding of the concepts presented.
- If time permits, address any other questions the students may have.

Lesson Plan / SAFETY

Anticipatory Set

Review previous lesson if applicable.

Bring samples of items that are used for safety (bike helmet, mouth guard, shin guards, goggles, seat belt, safety signs, etc.)

Ask for examples (crossing at the green light, walking not running in the hallways, etc.)

Bring supplies to create an emergecy and dental emergency kit for school.

Objectives

Student will be able to name at least 3 safety rules.

Student will be able to name at least 3 items found in an emergency kit.

Students will be able to name at least 1 item that is used as protective equipment.

Instruction/Information

Visual: Present the dental safety rules or discuss the protective equipment/safety tips (4–6 grades).

Discuss the items needed to make up an emergency kit for home or school.

Discuss the items used for a dental emergency.

Guided Practice Activities

Hold up samples of items and ask if they agree or disagree if the item is a safty or protective equipment that should be used (thumbs up or down).

Create an emergency kit and/or a dental emergency kit for school.

Closure

1. Name at least 3 safety rules.

2. Name at least 1 or more items used for a dental emergency.

3. Give examples of protective equipment or a safety tip.

NAME _____

List the items that would be in your Dental Emergency Kit.

1. _____

2. _____

3. _____

4. _____

5. _____

6. _____

7. _____

8. _____

9. _____

10. _____

11. _____

12. _____

NAME _____

List the safety rules that you will follow.

1. _____

2. _____

3. _____

4. _____

5. _____

6. _____

7. _____

8. _____

9. _____

10. _____

Figure 10–1   Dental Emergency Worksheet.

Play safe

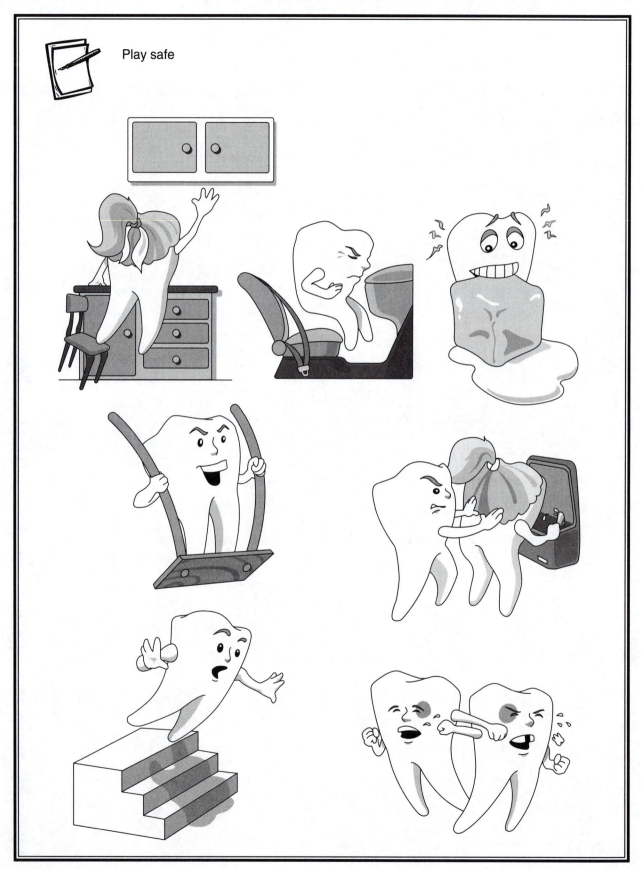

FIGURE 10–2 Play It Safe.

CHAPTER 11

Anti-Tobacco Lessons

Note: Check with the school administration for specific protocols if you plan to bring any tobacco products onto school grounds.

PREPARATION

(5 minutes before beginning lesson)

Display different pictures of forms of tobacco and tobacco products: cigarettes, cigars, pipe tobacco, and smokeless tobacco (snuff, chewing tobacco).

ANTICIPATORY PLANNING

(5 minutes)

- Review the previous lesson, if applicable.
- Introduce presenters.
- Describe the goals of today's lesson, the format of information, and general topics to be covered.
- Review classroom rules (K–3), if applicable.
- Survey the class's tobacco exposure or awareness. (Ask: How many know of someone who uses smokeless tobacco or any form of tobacco?)

General Objectives by Grade Level

(2–3 minutes)

State specifically not more than three objectives appropriate for the classroom learning level that indicate what the majority of the students will be able to achieve by the completion of the lesson. Keep in mind that for every grade level you advance, the previous grade level objectives could also be used.

Upon completion of this lesson, the student will be able to achieve the objectives listed in the following table.

GR	OBJECTIVE
K	Distinguish between good and bad habits.
	Distinguish between good and bad air flow.
	Identify tobacco as a bad habit.
	Relate healthy lungs to breathing and air supply.
1	List three ways one can protect oneself from side stream and secondary smoke.
2	Identify at least three parts of the body directly affected by tobacco use.
	Describe the possible effects of tobacco use on those parts.
3	Describe smokeless tobacco.
	Recognize smokeless tobacco as an unsafe alternative to cigarette smoking.

(continued)

GR	OBJECTIVE
4	Define peer pressure.
	State at least three ways to say "no" to using tobacco.
	Identify at least two tricks used by advertisers to promote tobacco use.
5	Discuss social- and health-related consequences.
6	Include any or all of the above information.

INSTRUCTION/INFORMATION

(10 minutes)

More than one topic may be included or combined with the guided practice segment (10–20 minutes). Use as many visuals as possible for grades K–3; group discussion may be more appropriate for grades 4–6.

- Discuss good habits versus bad habits.
- Show examples of or discuss the different types of tobacco.
- Use the handout illustrating Tobacco Tom's body structures to discuss the effects of tobacco.
- Discuss alternatives to tobacco, and alternatives to side stream or second-hand smoke exposure.
- Present the fact sheet about tobacco (see Appendix).
- Discuss the link between tobacco and oral cancers.
- Discuss social- and health-related consequences of tobacco use.
- Present your survey of the cost of tobacco products.
- Relate the advertising tricks of the trade used by tobacco companies to entice new smokers.
- Review the most common concerns students have about tobacco use.

Good Habits Versus Bad Habits

Begin the discussion by defining the word "habit" (a tendency to do something over and over again, without really thinking about it). On the black/white board, list good habits at home and school, as follows:

- Brushing and flossing your teeth
- Combing your hair
- Washing your hands
- Eating healthful foods
- Playing safely
- Raising your hands
- Sitting quietly in your seats

Next, list bad habits at home and school, as follows:

- Putting objects in your mouth (erasers, pencils, pens, paper clips, pins, and coins)
- Talking out of turn
- Biting your nails
- Twisting your hair
- Smoking

Use visuals to reinforce the discussion. Have pictures of the following items:

- *Good habits*: (1) brushing, (2) flossing, (3) fluoride, (4) eating good foods, (5) good dental habits.

- *Bad habits*: (1) dental decay; (2) sore, bleeding gums; (3) tobacco, tobacco plant, tobacco leaves, cigarettes, cigars, pipes, and smokeless tobacco; (4) stained teeth; (5) mouth sores; (6) unhealthy person

Use the following scripts to describe the good habit pictures you have provided and to discuss the benefits and consequences of their actions.

1. Brushing
   a. *Benefit*: Cleans teeth and gums and removes plaque so you have fewer cavities and less chance of bleeding gums.
   b. *Consequence*: Not brushing allows plaque to form on teeth, causing swollen gums and cavities.
2. Flossing
   a. *Benefit*: Removes plaque between teeth, helps to prevent cavities, and keeps gums healthy.
   b. *Consequence*: Not flossing has the opposite effect.
3. Fluoride
   a. *Benefit*: Makes teeth hard and strong and helps to prevent cavities.
   b. *Consequence*: Lack of fluoride leaves teeth without protection and more susceptible to decay.
4. Eating good foods
   a. *Benefit*: Makes teeth and bodies healthy and strong.
   b. *Consequence*: Eating too many sugary or fatty foods increases acids, which attack the teeth-causing cavities. It also builds fat in our bodies, making it harder for our hearts to work.
5. Good dental habits
   a. *Benefits*: Good strong teeth and healthy bodies.
   b. *Consequence*: Tooth decay and gum disease.

Use the following scripts to describe the bad habit pictures:

1. Dental decay is a possible consequence of not brushing, flossing, or using fluorides.
2. Sore, bleeding gums are a consequence of not brushing and flossing.
3. The tobacco habit: Ask students: Who knows where tobacco comes from? (*Answer*: The tobacco plant.)
   a. Tobacco plant: Tobacco is grown in many parts of the United States as a crop, just like fruits and vegetables are grown by farmers.
   b. Tobacco leaves are cut and dried, then crushed until they look much like coffee grounds. They are then put into tobacco products to be sold.
   c. Cigarettes, cigars, and pipes are lit with a match so they will burn, causing smoke, which is very dangerous to our bodies. The consequences of smoking include lung and heart disease.
   d. Smokeless tobacco is another kind of tobacco, also called snuff or chew, that is not smoked but instead is put in the mouth between the cheek and gums. Using any form of tobacco is a bad habit because of the dangerous consequences.
4. Tobacco stains the teeth. Also, snuff and chew users have to spit, because if they swallowed the juices, it could hurt them and make them sick.
5. Tobacco gives us bad breath. It can also cause sores and white patches that turn into cancer. It can make our gums sore.
6. Unhealthy person: Tobacco can cause two serious diseases, lung cancer and heart disease, that harm our bodies and can make us very sick.

Tobacco Tom

Tobacco Tom and the Effects of Tobacco

Tell the story about a boy named Tom. Talk about how his friends try to influence him to try a smoking a tobacco product. Use pictures or make structures out of felt and display them on a flannel board to illustrate how tobacco affects different parts of the body: heart (enlarged), lungs (clogs the air sacs, making breathing more difficult), eyes (red and puffy), nose (irritated), teeth (yellow and stained). An additional unpleasant effect is the odor (smelly hair, breath, hands, clothes, environment).

This discussion can be followed by a guided practice activity in which students use the handout provided at the end of this lesson to illustrate the changes that occur with tobacco use.

Alternatives to Smoking

Present the following healthy alternatives to smoking. Ask students if they can identify other healthy habits to replace smoking.

- Seek professional help from a dentist, dental hygienist, or physician about smoking cessation programs.
- Find a new—good—habit to replace smoking (e.g., eat carrots and other healthy snacks, chew sugarless gum).

Alternatives to Side Stream or Secondhand Smoke Exposure

Elicit from the class alternatives to staying in a smoke-filled room or other location by asking students what they would do if in that situation. Possible options include:

- Go into another room.
- Go outside.
- Ask the adult to please not smoke around you (explain that it makes it difficult for you to breathe, makes your eyes water, smells bad, etc.).
- Ask the smoker to go outside.
- Roll down the windows if in a car (Table 11-1).

Discussion: Smokeless Tobacco Fact Sheet

Present the Smokeless Tobacco Fact Sheet (see Appendix). Highlight the following points:

- A can of smokeless tobacco contains three times the amount of nicotine in one pack of cigarettes.
- Smokeless tobacco is a drug. It is as addicting as heroin or crack cocaine.
- A bug in a jar with a moistened tobacco leaf will die within a half hour from the toxins.
- The first time most people try smokeless tobacco, they get sick.
- The earlier the age at which a person first tries smokeless tobacco, the more likely he or she will become addicted.
- Within approximately six months of using smokeless tobacco, it is possible to recognize changes in the tissues of the mouth.
- The levels of bacteria in tobacco increase during the growth of the tobacco leaf, during processing, while it is on the shelf, and again in the mouth.

General Information: The Link Between Smokeless Tobacco and Oral Cancers

One estimate fixes the number of smokeless tobacco users in the United States at 22 million. Sales of smokeless tobaccos have increased by over 30 percent in the past 10 years, while sales of cigarettes, cigars, and pipe tobacco have declined. Industry analysts predict that the number of users could double over the

Table 11–1   Health-Related Consequences of Tobacco Use

Not Smoking Cigarettes	Smoking Cigarettes
Better health	Lung cancer
Able to taste food	Lung diseases
Able to smell	Cough
Breathe easily	Shortness of breath
More energy	Loss of stamina
Will not get addicted	More frequent illness
Greater endurance	Heart disease
	Addiction
	Dizziness
	Nausea
	Deadened taste buds/smell

Not Using Smokeless Tobacco	Using Smokeless Tobacco
Better sense of taste	Gum disease
Better sense of smell	Cancer of the mouth
Healthier gums	Cancer of the larynx
Fewer cavities	Decreased athletic performance
Will not develop a habit	Loss of teeth
	Addiction
	Tooth decay

next few years as health-conscious Americans look for alternatives to cigarette smoking.

Forms of smokeless tobacco include:

- Moist and dry snuff
- Loose-leaf chewing tobacco
- Plug or pressed-leaf chewing tobacco
- Hine-cut and twist chewing tobacco

Among the factors contributing to the growth in the numbers of smokeless tobacco users are the following:

- An increasing number of public places that forbid smoking
- Americans' increased participation in sports and outdoor activities in which participants need to keep their hands free
- The popularity of smokeless tobacco use among lifestyle and sports role models
- Weaning from cigarettes by former smokers
- The monetary savings of chewing tobacco compared with smoking cigarettes (A 3-ounce pouch of loose-leaf chewing tobacco can last a week.)

Smokeless tobaccos, which tobacco manufacturers claim are a safe alternative to cigarette smoking, actually contain high concentrations of certain carcinogens (substances that cause cancer) as well as 30 metals and a radioactive compound called polonium-210, and create a dependence on nicotine, as do cigarettes. Constant contact with a wad of smokeless tobacco (called a *quid*) can cause cancer of the esophagus, pharynx, larynx, stomach, and pancreas. Smokeless tobacco users are 50 times more likely to get oral cancer than non-users. These cancers can form within five years of regular use. Smokeless tobacco can also cause leukoplakia, a disease of the mouth characterized by white patches and oral lesions on the cheeks, gums, and/or tongue. Leukoplakia, which can lead to oral cancer, occurs in over half of all users in the first three years of use. Studies have found that 60–78 percent of smokeless tobacco users have oral lesions.

Nationwide, about 15,000 new cases of oral cancers are diagnosed each year, resulting in approximately 7,000 deaths. The incidence of oral cancer is almost three times higher in males than in females. Some signs of oral cancer include:

- Sores that fail to heal and bleed easily
- A lump or thickening
- Whitish patches
- Difficulty in chewing or swallowing food
- A sensation of something being caught in the throat

Other dangers of smokeless tobacco use include:

- Gum recession and increased sensitivity to heat and cold, resulting from exposed roots
- Drifting and loss of teeth caused by damage to gum tissue
- Abrasion of tooth enamel due to high levels of sand and grit contained in smokeless tobaccos
- Tooth discoloration and bad breath
- Tooth decay caused by varying levels of sugar added to smokeless tobacco to improve its taste
- Possible decreased athletic performance due to constriction of blood vessels caused by nicotine use

Advertising Tricks of the Trade

Following is a list of some common advertising claims or associations that are used to lure new smokers. Bring in ads from magazines to illustrate as many of these techniques as possible. Ask students to identify what tricks are being used to sell the product in each picture.

- "Amazing new product (or invention)": Stating that their brand is new and therefore better or more effective than others.
- Comparison: Comparing their "superior" brand to another "inferior" brand.
- Health appeal: Suggesting that their brand can do wonders for health.
- Sex appeal: Using beautiful women or handsome men to sell their brand.
- Symbols: Emphasizing a brand's logo or catchy saying.
- Bandwagon: Claiming that "everybody" is using their product and making you feel left out if you do not use it too.
- Having fun: Showing people having fun and implying that using their brand will help people enjoy themselves more.
- Mockery or put-down: Leading people to feel that they are doing something wrong or have failed if they do not use certain brands.
- Snob appeal: Claiming that rich people use their brand or saying that even though their brand costs more, it is worth it.
- Testimonial: Showing a famous person using a certain brand or talking about how wonderful a particular brand is.

Students' Most Common Concerns

Recite the following questions and concerns to the class, and ask if they have ever wondered about them. Follow each question or concern with the response indicated. Students may wish to address other questions or concerns as well. Be sure to involve the whole class and address everyone's concerns.

Concern: "My Little League coach uses smokeless tobacco and he is healthy (and older, wiser, my idol, etc.)."

Response: Explain that it is probably a habit with him. He may even be addicted. Review the meanings of these terms. Make the habit or the addiction the bad guy—not the person.

Concern: "Will my brother die if he keeps using smokeless tobacco?"

Response: Try to avoid using the word "die." The phrase "very sick" is better, but if you have to use the expression, say, "Many people who use smokeless tobacco don't die, especially if they stop using it. But, yes, some people do die."

Concern: "My mother smokes. I do not want anything to happen to her."

Response: Again, focus on the habit, not the person. Focus on how she will be getting healthier if she stops, not on the possibility of dying.

Guided Practice Activities

(10 minutes)

This segment may be combined with the preceding instruction/information segment. Visual aids are included at the end of the lesson.

- Have students label Tobacco Tom's body structures and show how they are affected by tobacco use (see Figure 11-1).
- Play the Lungo game (Table 11-2).
- Present the peer pressure group activity.
- Review various types of tobacco products, if displayed during the anticipatory or instruction/information segments of this lesson.

LUNGO GAME

Use the LUNGO card handout at the end of this lesson to keep score. On separate 3 × 5 cards, write out several questions and statements (true/false, multiple choice, fill in) regarding tobacco use, for example, Tobacco is good for your teeth: True or False. Or have students brainstorm questions to be asked and write them on the 3 × 5 cards. Next, assign a letter (from the word LUNGO) and a number (1–5) for each of the lettered questions as follows: L1, L2, L3, L4, L5, U1, U2, U3, U4, U5, N1, N2, N3, N4, N5, G1, G2, G3, G4, G5, and O1, O2, O3, O4, O5. There should be 20 cards each with an assigned letter and corresponding number on the same card.

Have each student draw a question from the numbered cards. If the question is correct, then the student blocks out or colors in the square on the scorecard that corresponds to the question number. The goal is to spell the word LUNGO by having five spaces in the same line blocked out horizontally, or to block all of the squares vertically.

The game ends when the first student achieves this goal. For an even greater challenge, have the students play until all the spaces are blocked out. Students can participate as individuals or teams.

PEER PRESSURE GROUP ACTIVITY

Divide the class into six groups. Assign each group a situation from those listed at the end of this section. Have each group discuss how they would respond to the situation. Share the answers and comments with the rest of the class (Table 11-3).

Table 11–2 LUNGO Game

	L	U	N	G	O
1.					
2.					
3.					
4.					
5.					

Table 11–3 Peer Pressure Group Activity: What Would You Do?

Group 1	Some friends form a new club and in order to become a member, you must smoke a full cigarette
Group 2	While sitting with a group of friends, the school's bully approaches and offers you a cigarette
Group 3	You are at a friend's house watching television, and both parents are smoking continuously. It is making your eyes water and you feel very uncomfortable
Group 4	At a ballgame, someone puts a wad of smokeless tobacco in his mouth and passes the package on to you
Group 5	You are sitting in a restaurant enjoying your meal when a person at the next table lights up a cigarette. Thick smoke is blowing into your face and stopping you from enjoying your food
Group 6	Your older brother or sister has just picked up a new habit of smoking and thinks it is very cool. He or she wants you to join in this new habit

Source: This information is summarized from CATS (Children Against Tobacco) workshop, sponsored through The Dental Health Foundation, Mary Maurer, M.Ed., and Tobacco Education,

CLOSURE

(2–3 minutes)

- Restate the objectives in question form.
- Check students' knowledge and understanding of the concepts presented.
- If time permits, address any other questions the students may have.

Lesson Plan / TOBACCO

Anticipatory Set

Secret word "Tobacco" write on the board and cover it up.
True/False quiz about the addictive aspects of using tobacco (4th grade).
Rolled-up fake cigarette with Supper Tooth coughing and gray clouds above his head (2nd grade).

Objectives

Identify three parts of the body affected by tobacco.
Describe possible affects to the body parts affected.
List three things about your personal appearance smoking will affect.

Instruction

Visual: Flannel-board story of Tobacco Tom's body and the tobacco effects (dirty clothes, smelly hair, watery eyes, etc.)
Methods: Lecture and class participation.

Guided Practice Activities

Tom's body matching body parts.
Discuss today's lesson with another family member.

Closure

1. Name one of the body parts affected by tobacco (ask three times).

2. Describe the possible affects on those body parts (ask three times).

3. Name one thing of your appearance that will change if you use tobacco products (ask three times).

4. Raise your hand if know what the secret word is (tobacco).

Independent Activity

1. Discuss this lesson with an adult at home.

NAME _____

Draw a line to connect: the words next to Tobacco Tom with the correct body parts.

Draw in the changes that occur in Tom's body when using tobacco.

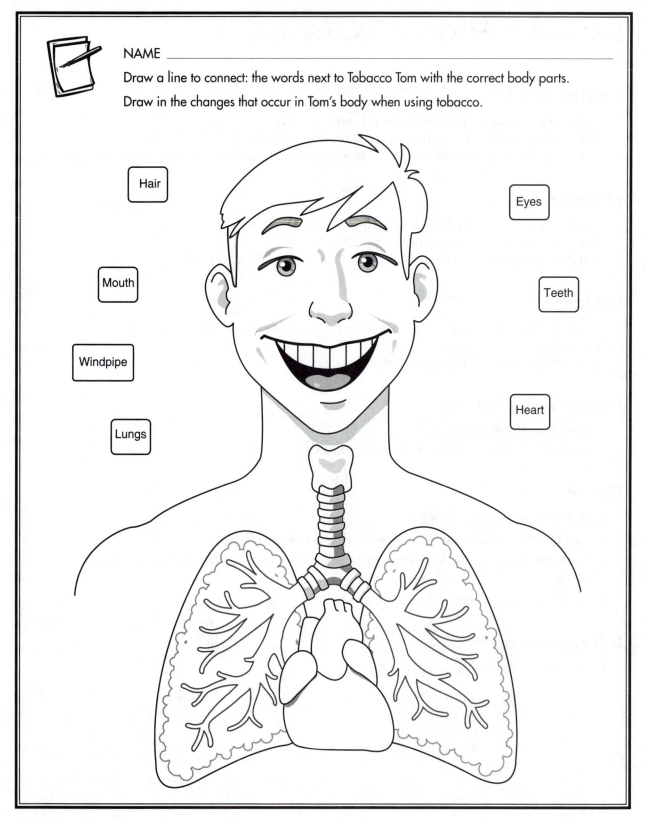

FIGURE 11–1 Tobacco Tom.

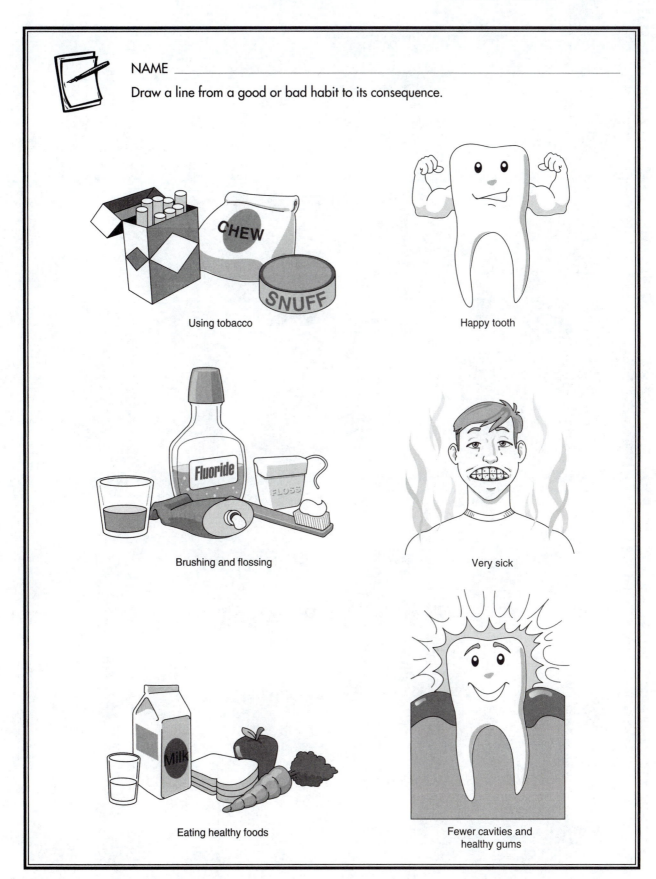

NAME _____

Draw a line from a good or bad habit to its consequence.

Using tobacco

Happy tooth

Brushing and flossing

Very sick

Eating healthy foods

Fewer cavities and
healthy gums

FIGURE 11–2   Health Habits Question.

CHAPTER 12

The Dental Office Visit

PREPARATION

(5 minutes before beginning lesson)

Dress up as a member of the dental health team; post large charts listing all the names and functions of the dental health team members; bring infection control gear; assemble the following items: a large tooth model and brush, tray of instruments, extracted teeth with fillings, sealants, and so on.

ANTICIPATORY PLANNING

(5 minutes)

- Review the previous lesson, if applicable.
- Introduce presenters.
- Describe the goals of today's lesson, the format of information, and general topics to be covered.
- Review classroom rules (K–3), if applicable.
- Survey the class about a few of their recent dental office experiences.

General Objectives by Grade Level

(2–3 minutes)

State specifically not more than three objectives appropriate for the classroom learning level that indicate what the majority of the students will be able to achieve by the completion of the lesson. Keep in mind that for every grade level you advance, the previous grade level objectives could also be used.

Upon completion of this lesson, the student will be able to achieve the objectives listed in the following table.

R	OBJECTIVE
K	Identify the importance of our teeth.
	Identify the members of the dental health team.
1	Describe instruments and equipment used in a dental office.
	Describe infection control procedures.
	Identify various duties of the dental health team in the dental office.
	Explain the function of a dental sealant.
2	Name and describe the functions of our teeth.
3	Relate the history of dentistry to modern times.
	Develop an appreciation for modern dental practice and procedures.
4	Include any or all of the above information.
5	Include any or all of the above information.
6	Include any or all of the above information.

INSTRUCTION/INFORMATION

(10 minutes)

Mote than one topic may be included or combined with the guided practice segment (10–20 minutes). Use as many visual aids as possible for grades K–3; group discussion may be more approriate for grades 4–6.

- Discuss the importance of teeth.
- Present the history of dentistry and review questions.
- Describe the members of the dental health team and outline their various duties in the dental office.
- Describe the instruments used in a dental office.
- Explain the importance of infection control during dental procedures.
- Discuss the use of sealants.
- Show diagrams of orthodontia problems and discuss their correction.

Importance of Teeth

Describe the parts of the tooth and the functions of teeth. Explain that teeth are used for (Figure 12-1):

- *Eating:* As we chew, our teeth help us cut, tear, and grind the food into small pieces. As the food is broken down, it is also mixed with saliva and the first phase of digestion is begun. If food is swallowed without being properly chewed, the stomach has to work harder and longer to digest it. This may give us a stomachache.
- *Talking:* Verbal: As air comes from our throat, it is caught with our lips, our teeth, and our tongue. In this way, sound becomes word forms. Nonverbal: The positions of the lips, teeth, and jaws also play an important role in making expressions.
- *Appearance:* Teeth help to form the face. Without teeth, the mouth sinks in and looks funny. Clean teeth give us an attractive smile.

Next, list the names and functions of the different types of teeth:

- *Incisors:* The four upper and four lower front teeth. The four central incisors are in the very front; the four lateral incisors are next to them. The incisors are used to cut food. They are included in both adult and primary dentition.
- *Cuspids:* The two upper and two lower corner teeth. The cuspids are used to tear food. They are included in both adult and primary dentition.
- *Bicuspids:* The four upper and four lower teeth next to the cuspids. The bicuspids crush and tear food. They are included in the adult dentition.
- *Molars:* The upper and lower teeth that make up the rest of the dentition. The molars are used to grind food. In the adult dentition, there are 12 molars; in the primary dentition, 8 (the first and second premolars) are replaced with the adult bicuspids.

Describe the parts of the tooth:

- *Crown:* The top portion of the tooth that is seen in the mouth.
- *Root(s):* The bottom portion of the tooth that holds the tooth in place. The incisors have one root; the bicuspids, one or two roots. The cuspids have one root, and the molars have two roots on the lower teeth and three roots on the upper teeth.

Tooth Tissues and Supporting Structures

Directions: Write the names of the parts of a tooth on the lines below.

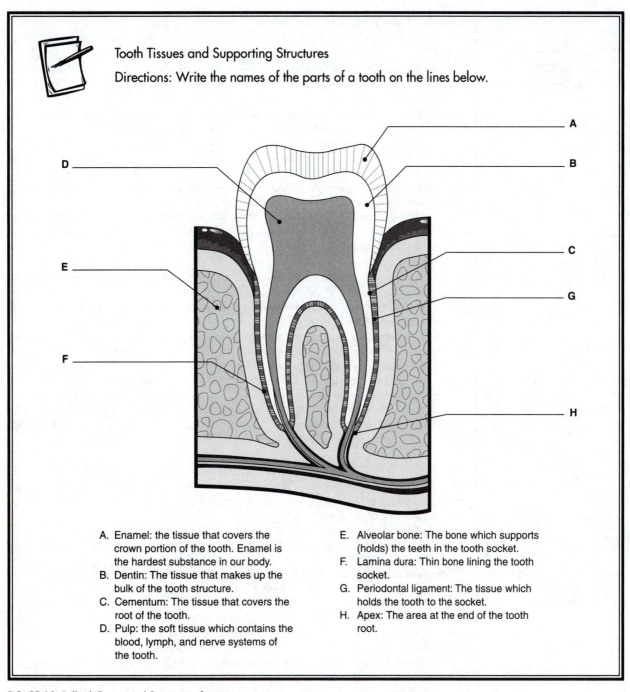

A. Enamel: the tissue that covers the crown portion of the tooth. Enamel is the hardest substance in our body.

B. Dentin: The tissue that makes up the bulk of the tooth structure.

C. Cementum: The tissue that covers the root of the tooth.

D. Pulp: the soft tissue which contains the blood, lymph, and nerve systems of the tooth.

E. Alveolar bone: The bone which supports (holds) the teeth in the tooth socket.

F. Lamina dura: Thin bone lining the tooth socket.

G. Periodontal ligament: The tissue which holds the tooth to the socket.

H. Apex: The area at the end of the tooth root.

FIGURE 12–1 Tooth Tissues and Supporting Structures.

**Story of
Dentistry**

The History of Dentistry

No one knows who the first dentist was or when he or she lived. It may be that the first dentist was a friend of someone who was troubled by a toothache, and that this person helped cure the pain by using a primitive chisel to knock out the tooth. For thousands of years, people blamed toothaches on evil spirits, so the first dentist may have been a medicine man or woman who practiced magic or the tribal religious leader.

Eventually, people began searching for something other than magic to relieve a toothache. They started experimenting with various materials and substances that they hoped would bring them relief. They tried herbs and offensive smells, which were usually aimed at driving evil spirits out. (Bad-smelling mixtures were thought to offend the evil spirits, thereby driving them out of the aching tooth.)

Dental knowledge has evolved slowly. It has taken thousands of years to reach the point we are at today. Here is how a dentist might have treated you if you had lived 250, 500, 1000, or even 3000 years ago.

- An Egyptian dentist might have advised a patient to treat a toothache by splitting a mouse in half and rubbing it over the aching tooth.
- A Greek dentist living in the fifth century B.C. would have used a mouse in a prescription for curing bad breath.
- A dentist living during the Middle Ages would have tried curing a toothache by having the patient inhale smoke. This is because dentists at the time were convinced that a toothache was caused by worms that got into the tooth. Thus, it was thought that fumigating the teeth with smoke would kill the worms.
- The early Chinese used arsenic to cure a toothache. It worked to a degree, because it killed the pulp of the tooth. However, the surrounding tissue would usually be damaged, which led to an abscessed tooth. As late as 1850, dentists in the United States also used arsenic to kill the pulp before they extracted a tooth.

Aristotle, a famous Greek philosopher who lived in the third century B.C., was one of the earliest people to associate sweets with tooth decay. "Figs and soft sweets," he said, "produce damage to the teeth, because small particles adhere between the teeth where they easily become the cause of putrefactive processes."

The Etruscans, who lived in central Italy from 1000–400 B.C., were the most advanced of all the ancients in the act of mechanical dentistry. They were very advanced in making crowns, bridges, and false teeth.

Roman aristocrats practiced restorative dentistry for esthetic rather than health reasons. They were interested in having false teeth to improve their appearance rather than as an aid to digestion.

Dentistry during the Middle Ages moved backward from where it had been during the Roman and Etruscan times. Barber-surgeons became recognized as persons with the skill to shave a man's face, cut his hair, extract his teeth, and perform minor surgery.

The Plymouth Colony brought the first dentist to North America about 20 years after the first Pilgrims arrived in 1620. His name was W. Dinley, and shortly after his arrival, he perished in a snowstorm as he was traveling to Roxbury to pull a tooth for a patient.

In April 1768, Dr. John Baker, the first competent dentist to practice in the American colonies, left Boston and went to New York. His advertisement in the *New York Journal* claimed that he could cure scurvy, fill hollow teeth with lead or gold, and make false teeth that looked as good as a person's natural teeth. (False teeth at that time were made from ivory, and they neither fit well nor looked as nice as natural teeth.)

One of our most famous Revolutionary War heroes, Paul Revere, was a dentist. The most famous false teeth in American history were those worn by our first president, George Washington. He had several sets of false teeth, but none were made from wood; rather, all were made from ivory.

The world's first dental school opened its doors in 1840 in Baltimore, Maryland. Until then, dentists got their training through an apprenticeship program, supplemented with whatever dental books were available. They had no background or knowledge of anatomy, pathology, or other related sciences. It took many years for the idea of a dental school to take hold. The changes in dental education were slow and gradual, but eventually the profession realized that a higher quality of training could be attained at a dental college than through an apprenticeship program. In 1859, Dr. Emeline Roberts Jones, a woman, began her practice in Danielsonville, Connecticut. In 1893, there were 150 woman dentists in the United States.

Today, all dentists must graduate from a dental college, then pass a state licensing examination before they can practice dentistry. This is one reason that history's most highly trained and capable dentists are practicing today. They are doing things that the dentists of the past could only dream about. They can treat and cure gum disease, straighten crooked teeth, and aid in the prevention of dental disease.

Follow-up Discussion: The History of Dentistry

Have students address the following points as a follow-up to the story:

- Describe what it would be like to go to a dentist who lived 150 years ago.
- Are we caring for our teeth today in ways that people living 50–100 years from now will find strange?
- For the first time in history, we can prevent dental disease. Explain how.
- Compare opportunities for women in dentistry (dentist) and men in dental hygiene.

Members of the Dental Health Team

Describe members of the dental health team and explain their roles:

- *Dentist (DDS or DMD):* A licensed professional who examines the teeth for decay; prepares and fills the teeth with sealants, fillings, crowns, bridges, partials, or dentures; and performs extractions and localized surgery. A dentist may clean the teeth or delegate this to a registered or licensed dental hygienist.
- *Registered or Licensed Dental Hygienist (RDH/LDH):* A licensed professional who examines the teeth for decay; cleans and polishes the teeth; takes and processes the radiographs (X-ray pictures); applies fluoride and sealants to protect the teeth; gives oral hygiene instructions; and provides nutritional counseling. The RDH/LDH may also sterilize the instruments. (Note: Duties may vary in each state.)
- *Registered or Certified Dental Assistant (RDA CDA):* A licensed professional who assists the dentist, hygienists, or front office personnel before, after, or during the dental procedure. Like the RDH/LDH, the RDA may take and process the radiographs, give oral hygiene instructions, provide nutritional counseling, polish the teeth, and apply fluoride. The registered dental assistant may also be responsible for sterilizing the instruments. (*Note:* Duties may vary in each state.)
- *Dental Assistant (DA):* A professional who assists the dentist, hygienists, or front office personnel before, after, or during the dental procedure. The DA may take and process the radiographs, give oral hygiene instructions, and provide nutritional counseling. The DA may also sterilize the instruments. Some assistants are specially trained and licensed to work in various dental specialty offices (described below). (Note: Duties may vary in each state.)
- *Front office person:* A professional who greets the patients, assists them in making appointments, handles billing and insurance forms, and processes information into the computer. This person may also assist with the dental procedures as needed.
- *Dental Laboratory Technician (DLT):* A professional specially trained to make the crowns, bridges, partials, and dentures for patients in a dental office.

Some dental laboratory technicians work in a dental office; others have their own separate offices.

Discuss the different types of dental specialty offices:

- *Dental Public Health:* The branch of dentistry that deals with the community and public health of dentistry as its practice.
- *Endodontics:* The branch of dentistry concerned with diagnosis, treatment, and prevention of diseases of the dental pulp and its surrounding tissues.
- *Oral/Maxillofacial Surgeon:* The branch of dentistry that deals with extraction and reconstruction of the jaw.
- *Orthodontics:* The branch of dentistry that deals with prevention and correction of irregularities of the teeth.
- *Pedodontics:* The branch of dentistry that deals with the care of children's teeth.
- *Periodontics:* The branch of dentistry that deals with the treatment of diseases of the tissues surrounding the teeth.
- *Prosthodontics:* The branch of dentistry that deals with the construction, making, and fitting of artificial teeth.

Dental Instruments

Bring in several of the instruments used in a dental office (mounting them on a tray for visibility). Explain the use of each instrument.

- Mouth mirror: used to see the teeth
- Explorer: used to count the teeth
- Curet/scaler: a small pick used to clean teeth
- Prophy-angle/cup: used to polish teeth
- Vacuum tip: used to remove excess water from the mouth
- Fluoride tray: used to put fluoride on the teeth

Discuss the other equipment that patients would find: an X-ray machine, lead apron, air-water syringe, dental chair, and hand piece.

ORTHODONTIC PROBLEMS

Refer to Figure 12-3, which illustrates three common orthodontic problems: crowded teeth, overbite, and crossbite. Discuss the following problems associated with misaligned teeth:

- Cause problems with speaking
- Interfere with chewing and, therefore, lead to improper food selection
- Put a strain on the jaws and muscles leading to jaw pain
- Cause facial deformities leading to emotional and psychological problems
- Make it difficult to brush and floss, especially when teeth are tightly spaced
- Allow plaque to accumulate, leading to tooth decay, gum disease, and bone loss
- Lead to a poor self-image

Infection Control

Dress up with all the protective OSHA (Occupational Safety and Health Administration) gear and ask the class why we wear this in the dental office. (*Answer:* To prevent the spread of germs from one person to another.) Discuss the importance of washing your hands before eating, after using the toilet, and so on to remove any germs. Define *germs.* Explain that several steps are taken in the dental office to protect the dental office personnel and the patient from catching any germs. Protective gear includes:

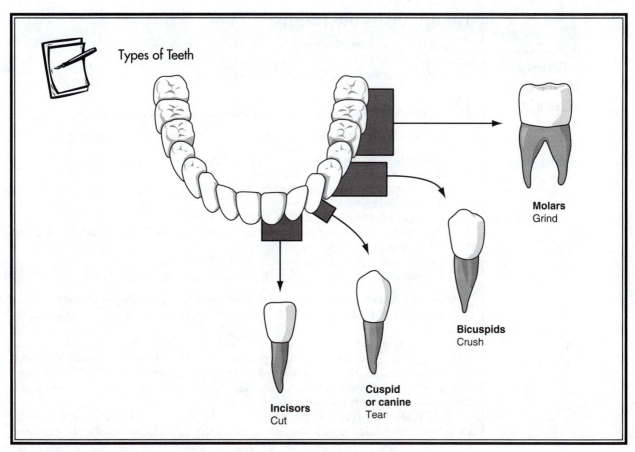

FIGURE 12–2 **Roles of teeth**

- Eye wear: to protect our eyes from splatter
- Mask: to protect our mouth and nose
- Long gowns: to protect our bodies
- Gloves: to protect our hands

Explain that barriers are placed over the dental operatory (the chair, light, hand piece, etc.) to protect us from germs, and that sterilizers are used to kill the germs on dental instruments.

Guided Practice Activities

(10 minutes) This segment may be combined with the preceding instruction/information segment. Visual aids are included at the end of the lesson.

- Relate the play or story Timmy Visits the Dentist.
- Present the comparisons of animal teeth.
- Many books are available about the visit to the dentist; provide a list to students (see Section 4).

Timmy Visits the Dentist

The goals of this activity are to encourage children to ask their school nurse for help if they are in pain, to acquaint them with the personnel in the dental office, and to familiarize them with dental procedures.

Place chairs in the front of the room for each of the characters to sit on.

ACTORS AND PROPS:

Timmy: a notebook, book bag, backpack, or lunch box
Teacher: a ruler, chalk, or pointer
School nurse: Red Cross arm badge
Timmy's father: necktie
Receptionist: phone, magazine (for Timmy's father)
Assistant: lab coat, bib clip, bib, tray of instruments, prophy cup, paste, fluoride tray, gauze, and saliva ejector
Dentist: white shirt, gloves, mask, and X-ray film in pocket
Hygienist: lab coat, mask, gloves, Typodont (large tooth model), brush

After the actors are chosen and dressed appropriately, explain the reason for the masks and gloves (to avoid sharing germs). Encourage the actors to do a little speaking during the reading of the story.

Once upon a time there was a boy named Timmy who was a student at _____ school. (Fill in appropriate name.) His teacher was named Mr. Gonzales. One day, as Mr. Gonzales was about to put the spelling words on the board, he noticed Timmy sitting in the front row looking very, very sad. He asked Timmy what was wrong, and Timmy said he had a terrible toothache.

Mr. Gonzales sent Timmy to the school nurse. The nurse took a look at Timmy's tooth and told him he needed to go to the dentist. When she called Timmy's father, he explained that the family had no dentist and they did not have a lot of money, nor did they have a car to drive to a dental office. The nurse offered to try to find a dentist in their neighborhood that they could walk to and one that would let them pay some money each month until the bill was paid. The nurse gave Timmy's father a number to call.

Timmy's father called the dentist, and the receptionist said to come right in. Timmy's father picked him up at school, and they walked to the dental office. At the office, the receptionist asked Timmy's father to sit in the waiting room and she gave him some forms to fill out and a magazine to read.

Soon the assistant came out to the waiting room and called Timmy's name. She took him into the operatory and put a bib on him. Next, she took an X-ray of the painful tooth. She went into a dark room to develop the X-ray, which she gave to the dentist. Then she took Timmy into the dentist's operatory.

The dentist checked Timmy's tooth and looked at the X-ray. Next, he put the tooth to sleep, removed the decay, and put a silver filling in the tooth. Afterward, the assistant took Timmy into the dental hygienist's room, where she cleaned his teeth using a tray of some special instruments, polished the teeth, and put fluoride on them. The dental hygienist reviewed toothbrushing and flossing instructions with Timmy.

At the end of the visit, as Timmy and his father left he dental office, the receptionist told Timmy to come back in 6 months for a checkup and teeth cleaning.

Follow-up Activities: Timmy Visits the Dentist

- Have students describe the duties of the dentist, receptionist, assistant, and hygienist.
- Have students name at least three instruments used in the dental office.

Animal Teeth Comparisons

If possible, bring in actual teeth to illustrate the differences between animal and human teeth. Or, bring pictures of as many different types of teeth (human or animal) as possible. Use diagrams to show how the shapes of various animals' teeth differ from human teeth.

Possible Activities

- Compare the size, shape, number, and function of each animal's teeth to the human teeth. Discuss how they vary and how they are similar.
- Discuss what devices we use to do some things that animals' teeth do with their teeth (e.g., squirrel uses his teeth to crack nuts, we use a nutcracker).
- Discuss why humans' teeth are more likely to be decayed than animals, the major factor being the type of food that is eaten. (Humans eat a lot of sweet foods.)
- Show pictures of animals as you discuss their teeth or have the children draw the animal pictures.

Preliminary Discussion

Teeth are shaped and formed according to their function. We use our teeth for eating, talking, and appearance, whereas animals' teeth are generally used for eating, obtaining food, and protection. Let us look at several different kinds of teeth.

Tooth Structures

Refer to Figure 12-1, which identifies the major tooth tissues and supporting structures. (Note: Each structure on the list that follows is keyed to the illustration by letter; e.g., A = enamel; B = dentin, etc.) Describe each part of the tooth to the class:

(A) Enamel: The tissue that covers the crown portion of the tooth. Enamel is the hardest subtance in our body.
(B) Dentin: the tissue that makes up the bulk of the tooth structure.
(C) Cementum: The tissue that covers the root of the tooth.
(D) Pulp: The soft tissue that contains the blood, lymph, and nerves of the tooth.
(E) Alveolar bone: The bone that supports (holds) the teeth in the tooth socket
(F) Lamina dura: The thin bone that lines the tooth socket.
(G) Periodontal ligament: The tissue that holds the tooth to the socket.
(H) Apex: The area at the end of the tooth root.

This illustration can also be reproduced as a handout for students to label and/or color.

Human Teeth

Humans have two sets of teeth: 20 primary (baby) and 32 permanent (adult) teeth. The teeth have four different shapes, and they vary in size and shape according to their use. The front teeth (incisors) cut, the pointed side teeth (cuspids) tear, the flat side teeth (bicuspids) crush, and the back teeth (molars) grind. (Refer to Figure 12-2.)

Animal Teeth

Present several different examples from the following list:

- *Bird:* The bird has no teeth and cannot chew its food. Therefore, nature has made it so the bird can swallow its food whole. When the bird swallows its food, the unchewed food goes to a sort of storage tank called the *crop*. As the bird needs nourishment, the food passes from the crop to its stomach, which is called the *gizzard*. In the gizzard are pieces of gravel that the bird has swallowed on purpose. The gravel helps grind the food into tiny pieces so the bird's body can use it to be healthy. While this system works fine for the bird, we must chew our food well before swallowing it.
- *Beaver:* The beaver has four front teeth, two on top, and two on the bottom. They are very strong and sharp. These teeth grow about four feet each

year. However, they never look very long because they are continuously worn away. The beaver uses its teeth to cut down trees, which it uses to build a dam. Then, in the pond behind the dam, the beaver builds its home. The beaver's dam helps it catch food and hide from its enemies.

- *Elephant:* The elephant has two big front teeth that come out of its mouth. These teeth are called *tusks.* They weigh from 55–200 pounds and can be as long as 10 feet. The tusks are made of ivory, and the elephant uses them to eat and to fight its enemies.
- *Walrus:* The walrus also has two long front teeth called tusks that stick out of its mouth. Like the elephant's tusks, the walrus's are made of ivory. They are much smaller, though, usually between 14 and 26 inches long. The walrus uses its tusks to tear seaweed loose and to dig up clams to eat. They also help the walrus move along the ice and land, in much the same way that we use ski poles.
- *Whale:* Whales are the largest living mammals (warm-blooded animals that nurse their babies). Some kinds of whales have as many as 3,000 teeth in each jaw. However, they are only 1/8-inch long. Other whales have no teeth. Most whales eat very small fish and swallow them whole. Therefore, whales do not really need teeth.
- *Vampire bat:* The vampire bat has two upper front teeth that are triangular and project forward. The edges and tip are razor sharp, enabling the bat to cut into the skin of its victims and suck their blood, which it eats as food.
- *Squirrel:* The squirrel has very strong teeth. It uses its teeth to crack the shells of nuts so it can eat the nutmeats.
- *Snake:* The snake has many tiny sharp teeth that help it swallow its food. The snake's mouth can be stretched to several times its normal size in order to swallow large animals. Many poisonous snakes have two long upper front teeth, called *fangs.* They are used to bite and squirt poison into the snake's victims. These fangs are hidden under a flap of skin when the snake's mouth is closed.
- *Cow:* The cow has no upper front teeth, but in their places are horny pads. Therefore, the cow cannot use just its teeth to get food. To pull grass out of the ground, the cow must grip it between the bottom teeth and the upper horny pads and then jerk its head back. The cow's back teeth are very flat. This is because the cow chews its food all day long and wears the teeth down.
- *Dog:* The dog has 42 strong teeth, including two upper teeth called *canine* or *eyeteeth.* These teeth are very sharp and pointed. The dog uses these teeth to fight its enemies and to tear meat into smaller pieces that it can eat.
- *Cat:* The cat has 29 or 30 teeth. It also has canine or eyeteeth similar to those of the dog.
- *Ape:* The ape's teeth are the most similar to those of humans. Both the ape and the human have 32 teeth. However, the ape's jaw is longer, and it has two very pointed teeth in each jaw.

CLOSURE

(2–3 minutes)
- Restate the objectives in question form.
- Check students' knowledge and understanding of the concepts presented.
- If time permits, address any other questions the students may have.

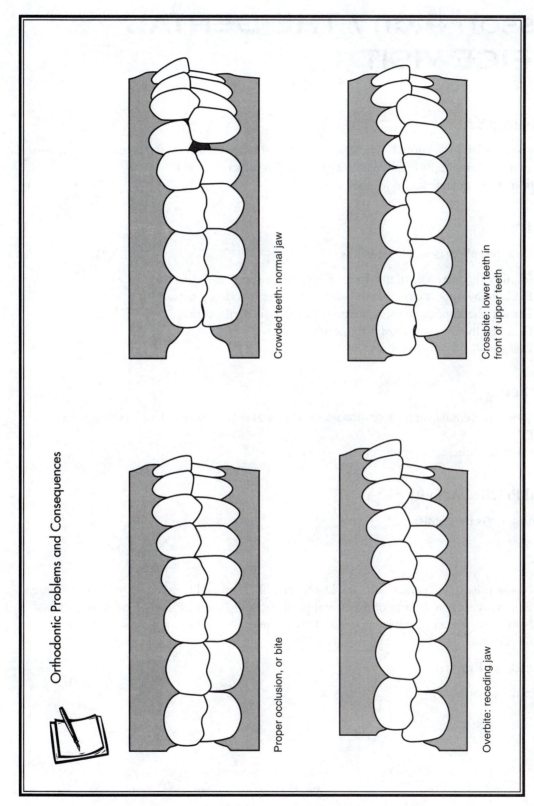

Orthodontic Problems and Consequences

Crowded teeth: normal jaw

Crossbite: lower teeth in front of upper teeth

Proper occlusion, or bite

Overbite: receding jaw

FIGURE 12–3 Orthodontic Problems and Consequences.

Lesson Plan / THE DENTAL OFFICE VISIT

Anticipatory Set

Pictures of health professionals working in the dental office posted on the board, dress in personal protective equipment (PPE; gown, mask glasses, gloves, scrubs, etc.)
Question? Does anyone know who we are?

Objectives

Students will be able to (select 3 objectives):

1. Identify the members of the dental health team and there education.
2. Explain the importance of each dental team member doing there job.
3. Explain the importance of infection control in the dental office.
4. Describe the importance of orthodontics.
5. Describe the tooth structures.

Instruction

Visual: Posters of dental health professionals, educational requirements, dental instruments, xrays, PPE.
Methods: Lecture, questions, group participation.

Guided Practice Activity

Play Timmy visits the dentist.

Closure

1. Name at least one person from the Dental Health Team and there educational requirements.
2. State why it is important for the dental professional to wear PPE when treating patients.
3. Name one reason why it is important for each member of the dental team to do there job.

Independent Practice

Visit your dental office.

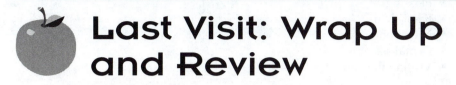

CHAPTER 13

Last Visit: Wrap Up and Review

PREPARATION

(5 minutes before beginning lesson)

Assemble a big tooth model, toothbrush, and other items needed for the lesson.

ANTICIPATORY PLANNING

(5 minutes)

- Introduce presenters.
- Describe the goals of today's lesson, the format of information, and general topics to be covered.
- Review classroom rules (K–3), if applicable.

General Objectives by Grade Level

(2–3 minutes)

State specifically not more than three objectives appropriate for the classroom learning level that indicate what the majority of the students will be able to achieve by the completion of the lesson. Keep in mind that for every grade level you advance, the previous grade level objectives could also be used. In this lesson, take the opportunity to check for knowledge and restate a variety of objectives previously given to the class.

Upon completion of this lesson, the student will be able to perform the following objectives and respond appropriately for his or her grade level:

- Describe the process of dental disease and its consequences.
- State how to prevent dental disease by toothbrushing, flossing, using fluoride, eating healthful snacks and food, eating sugar in moderation, using sealants, and visiting the dentist.

INSTRUCTION/INFORMATION

(10 minutes)

More than one topic may be included or combined with the guided practice segment (10–20 minutes). Use as many visuals as possible for grades K–3; group discussion may be more appropriate for grades 4–6.

- Review the information that has been given during the year.
- Present the typical review questions to test students' knowledge.

Review of Information

Review the information presented in previous lessons with emphasis on the following areas:

- Plaque control
- Prevention of dental diseases

- Toothbrushing
- Flossing
- Fluoride use
- Nutrition
- Dental sealants
- Visiting the dentist

Typical Review Questions

The following review questions can be used to tests students' understanding of the information that has been presented throughout the year. They can also be used with the Tooth-Tac-Toe, Stop the Pirates, and Blackboard Football games presented in the guided practice activities segment later in this lesson.

All Grade Levels

1. What is the sticky film that collects on our teeth after we have eaten food? (*Plaque.*)
2. How do you spell plaque? (*P-L-A-Q-U-E.*)
3. What does fluoride do for our teeth? (*It makes them strong.*)
4. How often should we brush our teeth? (*At least two times a day.*)
5. What happens if the plaque is not removed from your teeth? (*It forms an acid that can cause cavities or decay.*)
6. List two reasons why teeth are important? (*Possible answers: They help us to eat, talk, and look nice.*)
7. Name two things we can do to keep our teeth forever. (*Possible answers: Brush, floss, use fluoride, and eat healthful foods.*)

Grades 2–3

1. Name three foods that are bad for our teeth.
2. How do we get plaque out from between our teeth where the toothbrush cannot reach? (*By flossing.*)
3. Name two drinks that would be good for our teeth.
4. Name two sources of fluorides.
5. Describe at least one safety rule.
6. Name two places where the plaque likes to hide.

Grades 4–6

1. Spell fluoride. (*F-L-U-O-R-I-D-E.*)
2. Name three sources of topical fluoride. (*Toothpaste, mouth rinse, fluoride trays at the dentist's office.*)
3. Name three sources of systemic fluoride. (*Possible answers: Green leafy vegetables, fluoride tablets, fluoridated water, fish, tuna, fluoride drops.*)
4. Describe what you would do for a knocked-out tooth. (*Put it back in, put it in milk, or wrap it in gauze, and see a dentist as soon as possible.*)
5. List two specifications for a good toothbrush. (*Soft bristles, correct size for your mouth, straight and narrow bristles that are not frayed or worn out.*)
6. Describe the dental disease process. (*Plaque + Sugar = Acid; Acid + Healthy Tooth = Decay.*)

Guided Practice Activities

(10 minutes)   This segment may be combined with the preceding instruction/information segment. Visual aids are included at the end of the chapter.

- Play the Tooth-Tac-Toe game (grades K–6) (Figure 13-1).
- Play the Stop the Pirates game (grades K–6).
- Have the students find five things that will keep their teeth healthy (grades K–3).
- Give a quiz or post-test to check students' dental IQ (grades 2–6) (Figure 13-3).
- Play the Tooth Sleuth game (grades 2–6) (Figure 13-4).
- Play Blackboard Football (grades 3–6) (Figure 13-2).

**Trouble
in Open
Wide**

Trouble in Open Wide Melodrama

Introduce the characters (see Figure 13-5) and ask the students in the class to give a specific response when each character is mentioned. For example, when you say Boss Plaque's name, the students should say, "Boo-hiss."

Choose four students to hold name cards. Each name card should have a character's name on one side and the appropriate response on the other.

CHARACTERS:

Cowboy Healthy Smile (hero): "Wow!"
Sheriff Smilin' Sam (hero): "To the rescue!"
Boss Plaque (villain): "Boo-hiss"
Deputy Fluoride (heroine): "Hurray!"

Today we are going to participate in a melodrama called Trouble in Open Wide. It's a toothful tale from the wild, Wild West.

Our story takes place in an old Wild West town called Open Wide. Open Wide is surrounded by the Lucky Lips Mountains. In Open Wide, there lived our hero, Cowboy Healthy Smile *(Flash card: Wow!)*. Now Cowboy Healthy Smile *(Flash card: Wow!)* was very useful, helping out at the Talk Shop. Cowboy Healthy Smile *(Flash card: Wow!)* was always eager to help say words and letters clearly. He loved to help with talking.

Cowboy Healthy Smile *(Flash card: Wow!)* also worked at the Eatin' Place. He was a very good muncher and cruncher. He was always ready to help out with eating. He also was happy to make a healthy smile. Why sometimes, Cowboy Healthy Smile *(Flash card: Wow!)* was so busy, he had to help with all three—talking, eating, and smiling at the same time!

One day our villain, Boss Plaque, *(Flash card: Boo-hiss)* crept into Open Wide on his icky-sticky feet. He had every intention of taking over the town and capturing Cowboy Healthy Smile *(Flash card: Wow!)*. Boss Plaque *(Flash card: Boo-hiss)* and his icky-sticky dudes were pretty quiet. Nobody could see them because they were very good at hiding. Why, they were so good at hiding, they were invisible! They waited for just the right time to attack. Was Cowboy Healthy Smile *(Flash card: Wow!)* doomed to be captured by Boss Plaque *(Flash card: Boo-hiss)* forever? Yikes!

Cowboy Healthy Smile *(Flash card: Wow!)* could sense that something dangerous was about to happen. He yelled for help! To his rescue came our hero, Sheriff Smilin' Sam *(Flash card: To the rescue!)* with his strong but gentle brush, Buster. Sheriff Smilin' Sam *(Flash card: To the rescue!)* used Buster to give Boss Plaque *(Flash card: Boo-hiss)* and his icky-sticky dudes the old brush-off. Buster was very good at busting up the plaque gang! But Boss Plaque

(Flash card: Boo-hiss) and the icky-sticky dudes were pretty tough. They knew how to hide from Buster!

They were tough, but not too tough for Sheriff Smilin' Sam *(Flash card: To the rescue!)*. No siree! He attacked the icky-sticky villains with a clever rope trick called flossing. With his flossing know-how, Sheriff Smilin' Sam *(Flash card: To the rescue!)* could round up those sneaky hiding critters and move them out!

Now Sheriff Smilin' Sam *(Flash card: To the rescue!)* did not leave Cowboy Healthy Smile *(Flash card: Wow!)* without extra protection. No siree! Deputy Fluoride *(Flash card: Hurray!)* saved the day. Cowboy Healthy Smile *(Flash card: Wow!)* and the town of Open Wide were saved from another attack by Boss Plaque *(Flash card: Boo-hiss!)* and his icky-sticky dudes!

Follow-up Activities: Trouble in Open Wide

After reading the melodrama, ask students to:

- List the three functions of teeth.
- Describe the role of plaque in the decay process.
- Name three things we can do to help prevent decay. *(Brush, floss, and use fluoride.)*
- State the effects of fluoride on the teeth.
- Ask the students whether Boss Plaque will come back another time.
- Color activity (Figure 13-5) for melodrama characters.

TOOTH-TAC-TOE GAME

This game uses the typical review questions presented earlier in this lesson to test students' knowledge of the dental information presented during the year (Fig. 13-1).

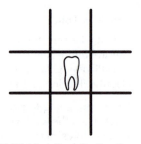

FIGURE 13–1 Tooth-Tac-Toe Game.

Directions

1. Draw a tic-tac-toe game square on the black/white board.
2. Divide the class into two teams, Molars and Incisors.
3. Ask the first player on the Molar team a question from the review list of typical questions presented earlier in this lesson. If the player answers correctly, then the team can draw a molar in a square of their choice. If the answer is incorrect, then no mark can be made.
4. Now it is the Incisors' turn. Ask the first player on the Incisors team a question from the dental review. Follow the procedure in step 3, but have the team draw an incisor in the square of their choice.
5. Continue the game until one team has a series of molars or incisors in a horizontal, vertical, or diagonal line on the board.
6. The teams can replay with different questions to finish the review of the lesson.

Suggestions

- Have the two teams use different colored chalk or erasable marker on the board, as the molars and incisors may look alike.
- For grades 4–6, substitute more difficult questions.

STOP THE PIRATES GAME

This game uses the typical review questions presented earlier in this lesson to test students' knowledge of the dental information presented during the year.

Directions

1. On the black/white board, draw five treasure chests on an island and a pirate ship off shore. Between the island and the pirate ship are five waves of water. The water is keeping the pirates from reaching the island and the treasure.
2. Divide the class into two teams, Pirates and Guards. The Pirates want to take the treasure, and the Guards want to hide it.
3. Ask the first player on the Pirates team a question from the review list of typical questions presented earlier in this lesson. If the answer is correct, the Pirates can remove (erase) one wave. If the answer is incorrect, then no waves can be removed.
4. Next, ask a question of the first player on the Guards team. If the player answers correctly, then one treasure chest can be buried (erased). If the answer is incorrect, then no chests can be buried.
5. The game continues until the Pirates remove the five waves of water or the Guards bury the five treasure chests.

Suggestions

- Use colored chalk or erasable markers to draw the picture on the board.
- For grades 4–6, add more waves and more treasure chests, and substitute more difficult questions.

DENTAL IQ QUIZ

Using the quiz handout at the end of this lesson, test students' knowledge of the dental information presented during the year.

TOOTH SLEUTH GAME

Have students use the tooth sleuth handout at the end of this lesson to discover individuals in the classroom who follow good dental practices.

BLACKBOARD FOOTBALL GAME

This game uses the typical review questions presented earlier in this lesson to test students' knowledge of the dental information presented during the year (Fig.13-2).

Directions

1. Draw a football field on the black/white board. Mark a goal post at either end and indicate the various yard lines (10, 20, 30, 40, 50, 40, 30, 20, and 10). Draw a football on the 50-yard line.
2. Divide the class into two teams (e.g., the Haunted Mouths and the Buzzard Breaths).
3. Ask one of the Haunted Mouth players a question from the review list of questions presented earlier in this lesson. If the player answers correctly,

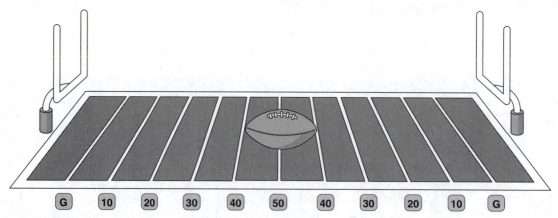

FIGURE 13–2 Blackboard Football game.

then the football is moved (drawn) so that it is on the Buzzard Breaths'
40-yard line.

4. Next, ask a Buzzard Breath player a question. If the player answers correctly,
   the ball is pushed back 10 yards to the 50-yard line again.

5. If a player gives an incorrect answer, then the ball does not move.

6. The first team that reaches the opponent's goal line has made a touchdown
   and receives six points.

7. A scorekeeper can score the game as shown:

Haunted Mouth	Buzzard Breath
6	6
6	0
12	6

8. The game ends when all of the review questions have been asked.

Suggestions

Use colored chalk or erasable markers to draw the football field, football, and field
goals on the board.

CLOSURE

(2–3 minutes)

- Restate the objectives in question form.
- Check students' knowledge and understanding of the concepts presented.
- If time permits, address any other questions the students may have.

Lesson Plan / LAST VISIT: WRAP UP AND REVIEW

Anticipatory Set

Review last lesson if applicable.
Describe the goals and format for the day.
Bring a combination of samples from previous lessons to review.

Objectives

Describe the process of dental disease and its consequences.
Describe the methods to prevent dental diseases (toothbrushing, floss, fluoride).
Name at least one item that you have learned since we have been to your class.

Instruction/Information

Review importance of plaque control, the dental disease process, preventive measures, safety, etc.
Remind the students of the importance of regular check ups in the dental office.

Guided Practice Activities

Set up and conduct the melodrama: Trouble in Open Wide.
For younger students, tell a story instead of conducting the melodrama.

Closure

1. Name at least one effect that happens to your teeth when you don't brush daily.
2. Relate the importance of a regular check up in the dental office.
3. Describe at least one way that can have healthy teeth.

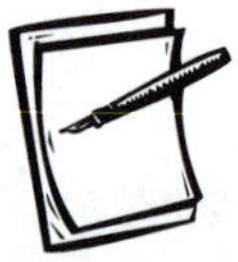

NAME _____

Dental IQ Quiz

Circle the correct answer (true or false) for the following questions.

1. You don't always need to take good care of baby teeth since they will fall out anyway

   True   False

2. Flossing your teeth is just as important as brushing them.

   True   False

3. It's important to eat a variety of good foods every day.

   True   False

4. You should brush your tongue daily.

   True   False

Circle the best answer for the following questions.

5. The best way to brush your teeth is:

   Up and down   Scrub hard   Wiggle jiggle

6. Which is a sign of gingivitis?

   Tooth decay   Missing teeth   Bleeding gums

7. A sticky film of bacteria that forms on your teeth is called:

   Plaque   Tartar   Gingivitis

8. Fluoride can be found in:

   Toothpaste   Toothbrushes   Crackers

Answer key
1. F 2. T 3. T 4. T 5. Wiggle jiggle 6. Bleeding gums
7. Plaque 8. Toothpaste

FIGURE 13–3 Dental IQ Quiz.

NAME _____

Find someone who. . . . . .

Quietly ask your classmates and teacher if they fit the description in any
of the boxes below. If they do, ask them to put their name in the square

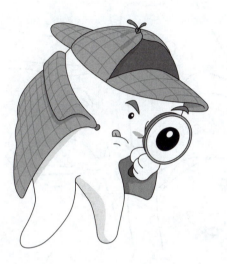

Tooth Sleuth

Find someone who has a cavity.	Find someone who has braces.	Find someone who has floss in his or her desk.
_____	_____	
Find someone who has fresh fruit in his or her lunch. (What kind?)	Find someone who eats a cereal that doesn't have any sugar added to it. (What kind?)	Find someone who brushes three times a day.
_____	_____	
Find someone who has been to see the dentist in the past month.	Find someone who is missing a tooth.	Find someone who uses a fluoride rinse at home (What kind?).
_____	_____	

FIGURE 13–4 Tooth Sleuth Activity.

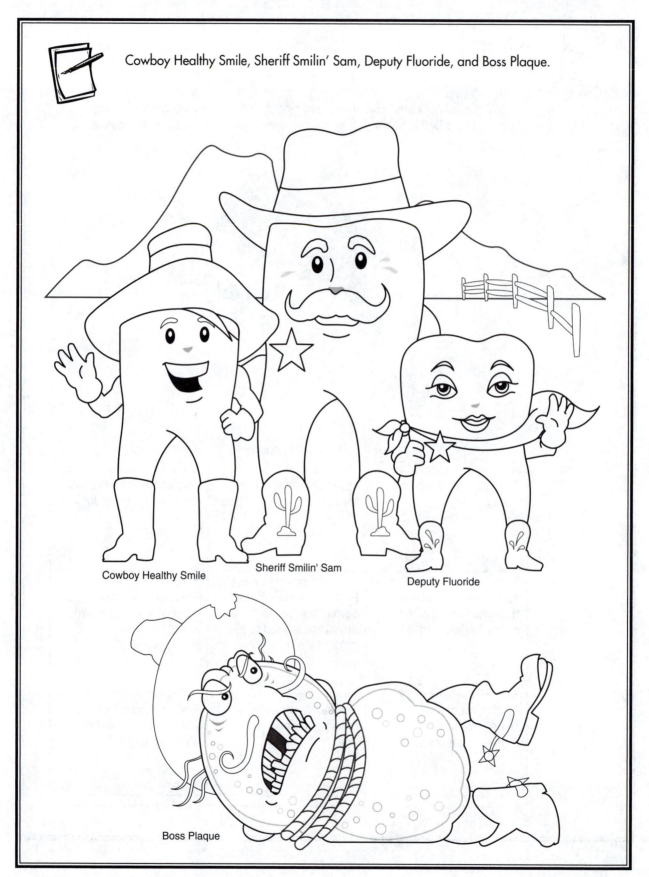

FIGURE 13–5 Cowboy Healthy Smile, Sheriff Smilin' Sam, Deputy Fluoride, and Boss Plaque.

CHAPTER 14

Children with Special Needs*

For legal purposes, pupils with special education needs should be designated "individuals with special needs." This designation should include only those pupils whose educational needs cannot be met by the regular classroom teacher with modifications of the regular school program, and who will benefit from special instruction and/or services. This chapter can serve as a reference when incorporating preventive education lesson plans into a classroom in which some or all individuals have special needs. The lesson plans presented earlier in Section 2 should be adapted and modified as needed to meet the needs of these learners.

The purpose of special education is to develop educational programs to help children with special needs to achieve the greatest possible self-sufficiency and success in the classroom. Dental health educators may encounter these children in the following settings:

- *Closed-campus programs:* The school's student population is made up of only special needs children ranging in age from 3–21 years who have various handicapping conditions. Most closed-campus programs specifically address the physically challenged child.
- *Self-contained classroom programs/special day classes:* The classroom is located in the regular school campus and may provide some mainstreaming opportunities for special needs students.
- *Mainstreamed programs:* Special needs children are integrated into the regular classrooms for the entire day. Modifications may be necessary or additional attention may be needed.

Several categories of special needs/special education classes may be provided in these programs, among them: autistic, developmentally delayed, hearing impaired, independent living skills, learning handicapped, physically handicapped, severely emotionally disturbed, and speech impaired. The following subclassifications may also be specified: communicatively handicapped, cerebral palsy, and severely handicapped.

The following suggestions are provided to help the dental health educator meet the needs of the special needs students in the classroom.

- Teach learning tasks in small steps, and sequence them in the proper order, one skill at a time.
- Check for knowledge at each step. Use repetition.
- If applicable, have students repeat orally what they have learned.
- Use different motivational strategies.
- Use a consistent and familiar structure when presenting information.
- Provide consistent reinforcement, especially in the development of new skills.
- Assess progress on a regular basis by checking for understanding and ability to perform the skills taught.
- Use visuals from the classroom such as puppets, toothbrushes, tooth models, etc., where possible.

- Provide continuous and immediate feedback for all activities.
- Invite caregivers, where applicable, to participate.

Dental neglect among students with special needs is often very high. The importance of dental care should be emphasized to caretakers, parents, and teachers. The remainder of this lesson presents information that can be used to improve the dental health of students with special needs. Use these suggestions when implementing the guided practice activities of brushing, flossing, and using fluoride in the classroom. Special positioning options are also presented.

BRUSHING

For the child with special needs, suggest that the teacher use the process of brushing to help meet other needs such as:

- Improving fine motor skills
- Teaching the parts of the mouth and their functions
- Improving language development
- Teaching self-help skills
- Teaching colors (Toothbrushes come in many different colors [red, blue, green, orange, yellow].)

The type of toothbrush and toothbrushing method should be geared to each individual's needs and ability (some have gripper or rubber ends to help with dexterity). Some students may not like having a foreign object, such as a toothbrush, placed in their mouths. You may have to work on desensitizing the child before thorough brushing can be accomplished.

Use a small toothbrush. Repetition and sequencing are very important. Emphasize the need to always start in one area of the mouth and end in a certain area to ensure that all areas have been brushed, and to instill the habit of thorough brushing right from the start.

When teaching step-by-step brushing, emphasize the steps in Figure 14-1.

If the child gags easily or cannot expectorate, then brush with a fluoride rinse instead of toothpaste. First, brush without the rinse. Then, pour a little rinse into a cup, dip the toothbrush into it, and brush with the rinse.

If total or partial assistance is needed, try to empower the child in some other way. Modifications or attachments may be necessary to adapt a toothbrush for a child with a physical impairment (see Figure 14-2).

FLOSSING

Only those students with the necessary coordination should participate in flossing. However, the importance of flossing should be covered. Emphasize that brushing is not enough. Flossing is needed to remove plaque between the teeth, where a toothbrush cannot reach. Daily rinsing with a fluoride rinse can give the child additional protection against cavities by strengthening tooth enamel.

When teaching flossing, emphasize the steps in Figure 14-3.

FLUORIDE

Depending on the fluoride level in the area's water supply, the appropriate method of fluoride supplementation should be used. If the child will not tolerate a fluoride rinse or tablet, then an alternative method should be tried. It may take a while before a child accepts the fluoride.

When teaching the use of a fluoride rinse, emphasize the steps in Figure 14-4.

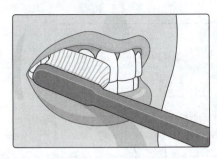

Place toothbrush bristles at the gum line, at a 45-degree angle to the teeth and gums. Press gently using short vibrating strokes, back-and-forth, or light "wiggle jiggle" motion. Start in the upper right quadrant at the last tooth, brushing the outside.

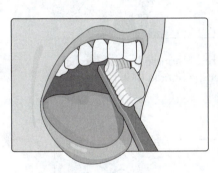

Move all the way around to the last tooth on the opposite side; then move to the inside and finish with the chewing surfaces. Do the same for the lower teeth. Be sure to brush each tooth.

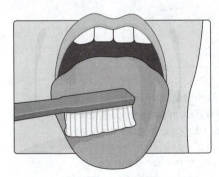

To clean the inside surfaces of the front teeth, both upper and lower, hold the brush vertically with the end of the toothbrush and bristles vertically at a 45-degree angle to the toothbrush and gums.

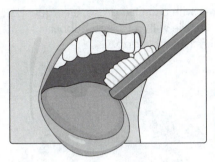

Don't forget to brush the top of your tongue, too, as it can harbor many bacteria. Move the toothbrush bristles with flat long strokes from the back of your tongue to the front end (stick your tongue out for this step).

FIGURE 14–1 Step-by-Step Brushing.

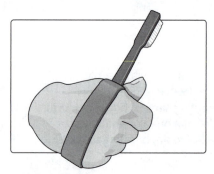

Attach the brush to the child's hand with a wide elastic band.

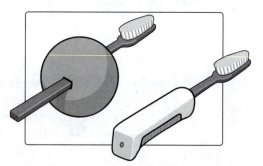

For children with a limited grasp, enlarge the brush handle with a sponge, rubber ball, or bicycle handle grip.

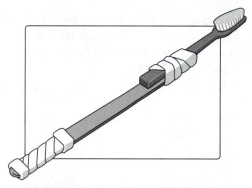

For children who can't raise their hand or arm, lengthen the brush handle with a ruler, tongue depressor, or long wooden spoon.

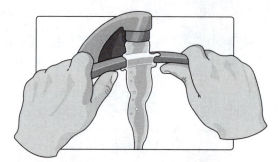

Bend the brush handle by running hot water over the handle (not the head) of the brush.

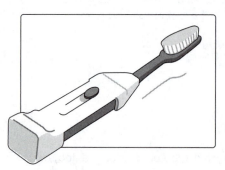

For children who can't manipulate a regular toothbrush, providing an electric toothbrush may enable them to brush by themselves.

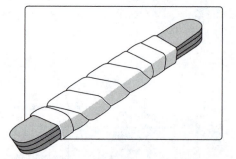

If the child can't keep his or her mouth open, use a mouth prop—for example, three or four tongue depressors taped together, a rolled-up moistened washcloth, or a rubber doorstop. (Emphasize that teachers and parents should always ask a dental professional how to use a mouth prop to avoid injuring a child's mouth.)

FIGURE 14–2 Methods for Adapting a Toothbrush. [Adapted from an original publication by Johnson and Johnson.]

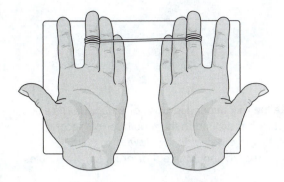

Take an 18-inch piece of floss and wind it around the middle finger of each hand. Or, tie the ends together in a circle.

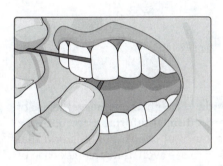

Grasp the floss firmly between the thumb and index finger of each hand. Hold a half-inch section taut for more control. Work it gently between the teeth until it reaches the gum line.

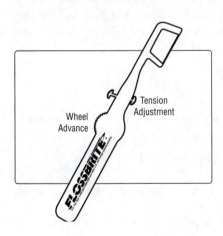

Curve the floss into a C-shape around a tooth. Slide the floss gently up and down the side of the tooth. Remove the floss gently and repeat for all teeth. Take care not to injure the gums with the floss.

A floss holder is highly recommended especially for anyone having difficulty guiding floss between their teeth.

- Flossbrite by Bergman Oral Care www.flossbrite.com
- Easy-to-use, single-handed flossing device
- Improved patient compliance
- Recommend for children, adults, and special needs
- Silk-like floss that glides through the contacts
- Disposable
- New floss and used floss rotates on separate channels inside the unit

FIGURE 14–3 Step-by-Step Flossing.

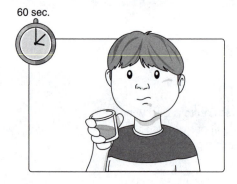

Have the child take the recommended dose of a fluoride rinse (usually a capful), swish it around in the mouth for 60 seconds, and then rinse out, taking care not to swallow it. To get full fluoride protection, the child shouldn't eat or drink for 30 minutes after rinsing.

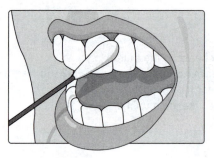

If the child is unable to rinse without swallowing, use a cotton swab or a toothbrush to place a little fluoride rinse on the child's teeth. The child's dental professional may also recommend a prescription fluoride gel treatment.

FIGURE 14–4 Step-by-Step Rinsing.

POSITIONING

If a caretaker is responsible for brushing the student's teeth, then review the use of alternative positions, which can make the procedure comfortable for both the child and the caretaker. Emphasize the importance of choosing a position that supports the child's head, allows the caretaker to see well, and ensures ease of manipulation during the procedure. If in doubt, then the caretaker should always ask a dental professional which is the safest, most comfortable position for the child. Emphasize the need to use care to prevent the child from choking or gagging when the head is tilted back (see Figure 14-5).

FINGER FLOSSING

Dental floss helps get your teeth really clean by removing plaque from between your teeth and under the gums.

1. Wrap about 18 inches of floss around your middle fingers.
2. Pinch an inch of floss.
3. Use your thumb and index finger to guide the floss between your upper teeth.
4. Use your index fingers to guide the floss between your lower teeth.
5. Work the floss gently between your teeth.
6. Bend the floss around the tooth in a C or U shape.
7. Now pull the floss against the tooth. Move the floss gently under the gum until you feel resistance.
8. Holding the floss firmly against your tooth, scrape the plaque from the side of your tooth, moving the floss up and down five times. Be sure to floss both sides of each tooth.
9. Move to a clean area of floss after every two or three teeth.

Place toothbrush bristles at the gum line, at a 45-degree angle to the teeth and gums. Press gently using short vibrating strokes, back-and-forth, or light "wiggle jiggle" motion. Start in the upper right quadrant at the last tooth, brushing the outside.

Move all the way around to the last tooth on the opposite side; then move to the inside and finish with the chewing surfaces. Do the same for the lower teeth. Be sure to brush each tooth.

To clean the inside surfaces of the front teeth, both upper and lower, hold the brush vertically with the end of the toothbrush and bristles vertically at a 45-degree angle to the toothbrush and gums.

Do not forget to brush the top of your tongue, too, as it can harbor many bacteria. Move the toothbrush bristles with flat long strokes from the back of your tongue to the front end (stick your tongue out for this step) (Figure 14.1).

Attach the brush to the child's hand with a wide elastic band. For children with a limited grasp, enlarge the brush handle with a sponge, rubber ball, or bicycle handle grip.

For children who cannot raise their hand or arm, lengthen the brush handle with a ruler, tongue depressor, or long wooden spoon.

Bend the brush handle by running hot water over the handle (not the head) of the brush. For children who cannot manipulate a regular toothbrush, providing an electric toothbrush may enable them to brush by themselves.

If the child cannot keep his or her mouth open, use a mouth prop, for example, three or four tongue depressors taped together, a rolled-up moistened washcloth, or a rubber doorstop. (Emphasize that teachers and parents should always ask a dental professional how to use a mouth prop to avoid injuring a child's mouth.) (Figure 14-2).

Source: Adapted from an original publication by Johnson and Johnson.

Take an 18-inch piece of floss and wind it around the middle finger of each hand. Or, tie the ends together in a circle.

Grasp the floss firmly between the thumb and index finger of each hand. Hold a half-inch section taut for more control. Work it gently between the teeth until it reaches the gum line. Curve the floss into a C-shape around a tooth. Slide the floss gently up and down the side of the tooth. Remove the floss gently and repeat for all teeth. Take care not to injure the gums with the floss. Flossing requires some degree of coordination and takes practice. It may help to use a floss holder (Figure 14-3).

Have the child take the recommended dose of a fluoride rinse (usually a capful), swish it around in the mouth for 60 seconds, and then rinse out, taking care not to swallow it. To get full fluoride protection, the child should not eat or drink for 30 minutes after rinsing. (Figure 14-4)

If the child is unable to rinse without swallowing, then use a cotton swab or a toothbrush to place a little fluoride rinse on the child's teeth. The child's dental professional may also recommend a prescription fluoride gel treatment (Figure 14-4).

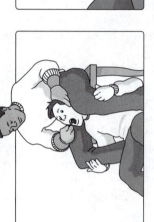

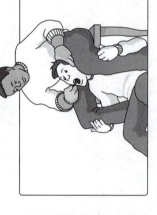

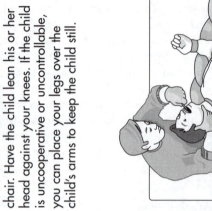

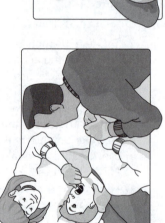

For the Child in a Wheelchair
Stand behind the wheelchair. Use your arm to brace the child's head against the chair or your body. Use a pillow for the child's comfort. Or, sit behind the wheelchair. Remember to lock the chair wheels first, then tilt the chair back into your lap.

Sitting on the Floor
Have the child sit on the floor, you should sit behind the child on a chair. Have the child lean his or her head against your knees. If the child is uncooperative or uncontrollable, you can place your legs over the child's arms to keep the child still.

Lying on the Floor
Have the child lie on the floor with his or her head on a pillow. You should kneel behind the child's head. You can use your arm to hold the child still.

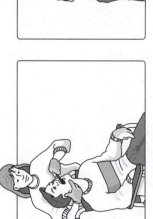

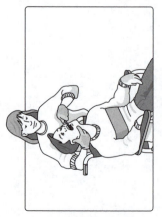

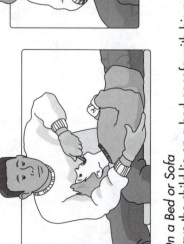

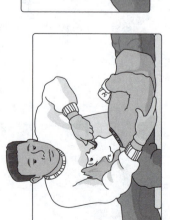

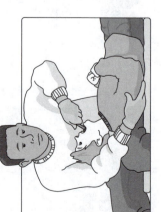

On a Bed or Sofa
Have the child lie on a bed or sofa with his or her head in your lap. Support the child's head and shoulders with your arm. If the child is uncooperative or uncontrollable, a second person can hold the child's hands or feet, if needed.

In a Beanbag Chair
For children who have difficulty sitting up straight, a beanbag chair lets them relax without fear of falling. Use the same position as for a bed or sofa.

FIGURE 14–5 Alternate Positions for Providing Dental Care.

Creating a Community Outreach Program

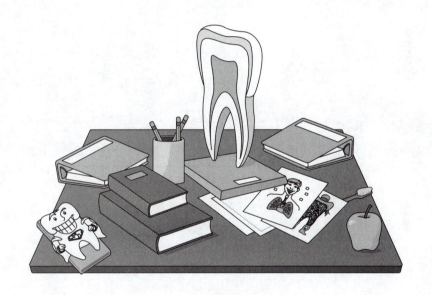

CHAPTER 15

Adult Learners

MOTIVATING ADULTS AND ADOLESCENTS*

Motivating adults to be better learners has been shown by research to make the adult feel more excited about what is learned, in addition to being more likely to put the new information to use. The first priority in providing an adult program with a high degree of motivation is to determine the needs of the audience. Pre-tests may be a valuable tool in assessing the specific needs of the group. Oral questioning may be another if the members participate freely and easily. Revision of the original outline may be necessary and changes initiated for the second and third visits if the group members voice needs that were not anticipated.

There is some conflict among theorists as to which of the educational domains are necessary in effective teaching. Some educators take a strictly behavioral approach, claiming teaching is no more than a transmission of facts. Some take a more humanistic view, feeling meaningful instruction must include both cognitive and affective elements. Still another view holds that effective teaching takes into account the attitudes, beliefs, and values, as well as the needs, of the learner. It should not be a difficult task to incorporate all of the stated theories into a three-part adult dental health program.

Attitudes are learned, are often deeply ingrained, and can be a major challenge to the educator. Every individual attending the dental health program will bring to that program different life experiences which will have had a profound effect upon the basic attitude of that person. In general, the more negative the attitude, the less motivation there is for change. Group attitudes can be very powerful. For instance, one vocal participant with a negative attitude can influence the entire audience. It is important to build upon and go with positive attitudes expressed by the participants.

In addition to need and attitude, highly influential factors in the motivational process include stimulation, competence, and reinforcement. Adults need to be emotionally involved in order to remain stimulated. Some learners may be stimulated by being told that they will be held responsible for answering post-test questions. However, be advised that some, especially those who have had little dental health background or have not have had their learning skills tested recently, may only be threatened by this approach.

Several different psychological theories concerning motivation hold competence as their central theme, supporting the idea that humans strive for understanding. Adults tend to be motivated when they feel a sense of accomplishment. The goal of the educator here would be to impart to the learner a sense of fulfillment and personal involvement rather than teaching only a particular skill to be mastered.

Reinforcement is necessary to facilitate retention and can be both negative and positive. Provisions for positive reinforcement should be built into the adult program at each step in the learning process. Motivation is sustained when the participant values what he or she has learned, enjoys the learning experience, and receives frequent positive reinforcement.

In order to achieve a highly motivational adult dental health program, the planning should include a series of learning activities based on the needs of the participants. It should be designed to specifically change behavior, emphasizing active participation by the learner, and a willingness on the part of the learner to take responsibility for change.

Source: Patricia Stewart, RDH, Ph.D.

Adult education is very different than working with students (K–8). Principles dealing with adult education, known as andragogy (the art and science of helping adults to learn), are based on core learning principles that include the following:*

- What it is and why the adult learners need to know the information.
- Self-direction by self-concept of the adult learner; being autonomous.
- Mindset from prior experiences (oral health condition in youth or current experiences that may be positive or negative).
- Willingness and readiness to learn something new or a new way of doing it.
- Learning orientation to a task-centered or problem-centered approach.
- Motivation of the learner (time involved, benefit, internal rewards, personal payoff, etc.).

When planning for an education program for adults or adolescents specifically state the goals and purposes for learning the behavior, keeping in mind the subject matter and individual differences. Adult learners are different from adolescents, seniors, and children; thus, teaching them can be challenging and will require a variety of teaching methods and strategies to keep their interest. To be successful in teaching adults, you will need to address the what and why adults or adolescents need to know the information, their readiness to learn, and the importance of motivating them to learn.

*Source: Summarized from: Wang, Victor, K. *Principles of Adult Education, A Guide to Optimal Performance in Adult Education.* Boston: Pearson Custom Publishing, 2003.

The following is a list of assumptions made about adult learners that applies to the principles of adult learners:**

- Adult learners want to see the immediate application of the material being taught to their own lives. Relate the value of good oral health to their appearance and their sociability. They will ask themselves, "Is this program worth my while?"
- Adults have knowledge, too. Most have had previous experience with dental care, etc. and they have "heard it all before." Be aware that they will want to share their experiences.
- Some adults will have made the choice to attend your program of their own accord; others will be attending your presentation in response to pressure from others. In any case, they will want to be sure it is worth their time.
- Adults may be shy. If it has been awhile since they attended any type of program, they may be apprehensive at first. Therefore, you may not get the adult learner to respond as rapidly as students.
- Adults will take direction; most are use to some sort of authority system.
- Adults really like to have fun. Create an atmosphere that is fun, warm, humorous, and friendly.
- Adults like to be liked. Give personal attention, compliments, etc.
- Adults are adults. Treat them like adults; they do not like being talked down to, embarrassed, or kept waiting.
- Adults are very social; they like to hear, share stories, and get to know each other.

** Source: Summarized from: Renner, Peter F. *The Instructor's Survival Kit.* PFR Training Associates Limited, 1980.

See Figure 15–1 for Adult Learner Evaluation Forms.

COMMUNITY DENTAL HEALTH ADULT LEARNER EVALUTATION

Please circle the number that best describes your feelings according to the following key:

4 = Met all our expectations
3 = Met most of our expectations
2 = Some improvement needed
1 = Little preparation exhibited

1. The presentation met the outlined objectives.   1 2 3 4

2. The presentations met the needs of the group.   1 2 3 4

3. The presentations were adapted to the group's level of understanding.   1 2 3 4

4. The dental information presented was effective.   1 2 3 4

5. There was opportunity for group participation.   1 2 3 4

6. The visual aides were effective.   1 2 3 4

7. The presentations were creative.   1 2 3 4

8. The dental hygiene students were able to maintain a high level of interest.   1 2 3 4

9. Please give at least one positive aspect of the presentation.

_____

_____

10. Please give at least one positive suggestion for improvement.

_____

_____

11. Please share any additional comments or feedback from the group.

_____

_____

_____

_____

Name of Evaluator _____

Thank you for your cooperation and participation.

FIGURE 15-1.

Low Literacy Learners

When presenting information to adults and/or participants with low literacy skills, it is essential to make your presentation understandable and acceptable. To avoid information overload during your presentation, the following four steps are recommended.

- Assess the participants' knowledge of their oral health condition and any risks that may be involved.
- Present new information instead of what they already know.
- Have meaningful interaction with the participants. Ask questions related to their responses.
- Outline the experiences they have had with their oral health.

The key in knowing what to expect is understanding the needs of these individuals. This will assure greater confidence and motivation for both the participants and the presenter. It has been estimated that 37 million people are uninsured and in need of access to the healthcare system. Many poor readers may benefit from your information and referrals.*

*Source: Doak, Cecilia Conrath, Leonard G. Doak, and Jane H. Root. *Teaching Patients with Low Literacy Skills.* Philadelphia: J.B. Lippincott Company, 1996; 151.

The Adult Lesson Plan

Things to be considered before you begin:

- How many visits will you make and how much time will you spend per visit?
- What content is to be covered at each visit?
- What are the characteristics of the adult learner population to be visited?
  - Sociological and cultural characteristics
  - Psychological characteristics
  - Learning styles and values
  - Experiences (past dental, etc.), interests, and educational needs of the adult learners
  - Stages of life (young, middle-aged or older adult, dependent/independent, etc.)
  - Physical characteristics (audio acuity, visual, dexterity, limitations, etc.)
- What skills need to be addressed so that the learner will become proficient in the instructional information?
- What are the instructional objectives?
  1. Are they reasonable to meet?:
     a. Performance (What should the participant be able to do?)
     b. Condition (What limitations are set of performance?)
     c. Criterion (How will it be done to be Proficient?)
- In what sequence will the objectives be taught?

Once you have considered all the above-mentioned information, plan your dental health lesson plan accordingly. Use the facts sheets (FAQ) as supplemental handouts during the presentations. You may want to survey the participants ahead of time to find out the type of information that would be of the most interest to these participating. Sample lesson plans of adult programs have been provided at the end of this section.

GUIDELINES FOR ORAL HEALTH PRESENTATION

The following is a list of topics to be presented. Fill in the time line as appropriate for your scheduled presentation. You may use all or some of the topics listed based on the amount of time and the number of times you can present information. Supplement your information with the fact sheets on various dental care topics found in the Appendix section.

Topic	Amount of Time
Plaque control	_____
a. Health dentition	
b. Etiology of plaque and calculus development	
c. Caries development	
d. Gingivitis and periodontal disease	
e. Disclosing solutions	
f. Bad breath/mal-odor	
Toothbrushing	_____
a. Manual	
b. Powder	
c. Types of toothbrushes	
d. Storage	
Flossing	_____
a. Flossing techniques	
b. Types of floss	
c. Floss hoders	
Care of prostheses	_____
a. Fixed	
b. Removal	
Fluoride	_____
a. Mouth rinses and gels	
b. Fluoride dentifrices	
Toothpaste (dentifrices)	_____
Auxiliary oral hygiene aids	_____
a. Proxy brush, rubber tip, perio aid, tongue scraper	
Antimicrobial products	_____
Whitening products	_____
Nutrition and its relationship to good oral hygiene	_____
Tobacco education	_____

Lesson Plan / ADULT PROJECT LESSON #1

Anticipatory Set

Arrive in scrubs carrying a big box of supplies, introduce yourselves and state why you are there. During the first lesson we will be discussing tooth brushing, flossing, fluoride, plaque, periodontal disease and nutrition.

Objectives

At the end of our lesson the students will be able to:
Demonstrate proper brushing and flossing technique with 80% accuracy.
State the primary cause of periodontal disease and two ways to prevent it.
State why tooth decay occurs and three ways to prevent it.

Visuals

Periodontal disease flip chart.
Typodont/assorted toothbrush ring.
Over-head transparencies of periodontal disease process & various types of caries.
Large foam tooth model.
Pamphlets: better dental health, senior care.
Samples: toothbrush, toothpaste and dental floss.

Methods

Demonstration: Proper technique of the Bass method and flossing.
Lecture: Plaque: what it is, where it is, what it does and how to remove it.
Decay: plaque/acid equation, how it occurs, how to prevent it and how to fix it.
Periodontal disease: what it is, how it occurs and ways to prevent it and keep it from progressing.
Fluoride: what it is, what it does and where it can be found.
Nutrition: why a well balanced diet is important, how certain foods promote tooth decay and foods that inhibit tooth decay.
Questions and answers at the end of every topic.

Guided Practice Activities

Proper brushing technique using the Bass method.
Proper flossing technique, wrapping of the floss around index fingers and creating a 'C' shape, hugging each side of the tooth.

Closure: (Questions)

Name three proper techniques for utilizing the Bass method/proper flossing technique.
Source: Jennifer Weitzel & Wendy Mertz Century College students.

Name the primary cause of periodontal disease and two ways to prevent it.
Discuss how tooth decay occurs and two ways to prevent tooth decay.

Follow-up

State what we will be discussing at our next visit, ask students to write down any questions they may have about today's lesson (to be addressed next time), and have students call their city's utilities department to find out if their water supply is fluoridated.

Lesson Plan / ADULT PROJECT LESSON #2

Anticipatory Set

Arrive in scrubs carrying a big box of supplies, reintroduce yourselves and state what you will be discussing today. Answer any questions that students may have had after the regarding the last lesson. During our second lesson we will be discussing baby-bottle tooth decay, periodontal disease associated with systemic diseases, common medications as they relate to dentistry, xerostomia, oral cancer/anti-tobacco, denture care, esthetic dentistry, safety and emergency care.

Objectives

At the end of this lesson the students will be able to:
State the cause of baby-bottle toot decay and at least three ways to prevent it.
State what xerostomia is and how to treat it.
Demonstrate how to do a self-oral cancer exam with 80% accuracy.

Visuals

Anti-tobacco poster.
Example of non-tobacco containing snuff.
Overhead of common oral cancer sites.
Various pamphlets containing information regarding baby-bottle tooth decay, esthetic dentistry and common medications that cause xerostomia.
Example of a product that is made to treat xerostomia.
List of affordable dental care facilities.

Methods

Lecture: Baby-bottle tooth decay: what causes it, how to prevent it and how to treat it.
Esthetic dentistry: various types of restorations and tooth whitening systems.
Systemic diseases: how they affect oral health, medications, and how they affect oral health, dental visit and xerostomia causing medications and how to treat it.
Tobacco/oral cancer: how smoking affects oral health, what causes oral cancers, how it is treated, how to prevent it, what to do if you suspect cancer, common sites for oral cancers.
Safety/emergency care: how to prevent accidents involving the mouth, what to do and where to go if having a dental emergency.
Demonstration: Oral cancer self-exam.

Guided Practice Activities

Oral cancer self-exam.

Closure: (Questions)

What is the primary cause of baby-bottle tooth decay and how could it be prevented?
What is xerostomia, what are some things that can cause it, how is it treated?
Where are the most common areas for an oral cancer to occur?

Follow-up

Let students know that we have pamphlets on the various topics that we have discussed and information regarding low-cost dental care that they are welcome to have. Answer any questions the students may have.

Lesson Plan / ADULT PROJECT LESSON #3

Anticipatory Set (Goals, Standards, focuser)

1. Teach proper toothbrushing technique for teeth and partials or dentures.
2. Instruct proper use of dental floss.
3. Education about the use of fluoride.
4. Teach basic information about plaque, bacteria, decay and periodontal health.
5. Discuss systemic disease as it pertains to oral health.

Objectives

1. By the end of the lesson, students will correctly demonstrate the correct techniques for flossing their teeth and brushing using the Bass technique.
2. By the end of the lesson the students will correctly relate two types of systemic disease to the importance of proper oral home care.
3. By the end of the instruction, the students will state three signs of gingival disease and inflammation with 100% accuracy.

Instruction (Methods)

1. Use a flip chart with pictorials to help depict the correct technique of toothbrushing using the bass technique. Do in conjunction with educators demonstrating on a large set of teeth, typodont, and in the mouth. Educate on using a soft brush, when to change brushes and different brush models. Display examples of different types of toothbrushes. Introduce plaque by putting shaving cream on the large wooden tooth model and remove it with a large toothbrush using the Bass technique. With a flip chart illustrate the correct technique for holding floss and using it in the mouth. Use a set of large wooden teeth and yarn to demonstrate flossing. Demonstrate the correct technique inside the mouth. Provide samples of different types of floss for students to examine such as dental tape, waxed, non-waxed, Gortex, and flavored. Discuss the correct way to clean dentures.
2. Discuss the use of fluoride and show examples of both tablets and liquid rinse. Demonstrate the use and reinforce the properties of fluoride. Provide examples of both types of fluoride for students to examine. Show a flip chart with a picture depicting a force field effect.
3. Use overhead transparencies to depict the stages of periodontal disease. Also show slides of patients at different stages of periodontal disease to reinforce tissue description and inflammation. Introduce terminology in both English and Spanish sing a flipcart. Display the large teeth models to show where plaque hides and the need to remove it efficiently. Also use a felt board to explain the "acid" equation of decay. Reinforce tooth brushing again.
4. The final topic is systemic disease, as it pertains to dental health. Explain by using a flip chart for terminology in English and Spanish. Emphasize the disease entities that class members have or members of their family may have, including diabetes and hypertension. Show a blood pressure cuff and sphygmomanometer.
5. The adult class instructor will translate as needed.

Lesson Plan continued

Visuals

1. Educator demonstration.
2. Floss and toothbrush samples.
3. Overhead transparencies.
4. Use of large teeth models and yarn, toothbrush, and shaving cream.
5. Flip chart with terminology in both English and Spanish, including pictures.
6. Slides depicting periodontal disease.
7. Demonstration of taking blood pressure.
8. Handouts to be given to students.

Guided Practice Activities

1. Students will participate in brushing and flossing their teeth and help will be provided when needed.

Closure

1. Review topics briefly and ask students questions regarding the objectives. Also, allow time for students questions.
2. Distribute handout regarding subjects covered in this lesson.
3. Distribute samples of toothbrushes, toothpaste, and floss.
4. Introduce the topics to be discussed at the next visit along with the day and time. Those topics include: reading food labels, baby-bottle syndrome, sealants, dental emergencies and safety, and tobacco.

Independent Practice

1. Encourage students to practice their new skills at home and to teach other family members.

Lesson Plan / ADULT PROJECT LESSON #4 DENTAL HEALTH FOR ADULT LEARNERS

Anticipatory Set (Goals, Standards, Focuser)

1. Review previous lesson plan one and answer any questions.
2. Teach students the importance of reading labels for good nutrition.
3. Educate students on baby-bottle syndrome.
4. Educate students on the use of sealants to prevent tooth decay.
5. Teach students the need for dental safety and the steps to follow if a dental emergency should arise.
6. Instruct the students on the dangers of tobacco use and oral cancer.

Objectives

1. By the end of the lesson the students will state reasons why reading food labels is important to good nutrition and name three good snacks for children.
2. By the end of the lesson the student will name one piece of safety equipment and correctly state the 5 basic steps taken in a dental emergency.
3. By the end of the lesson the student will correctly state three negative effects that tobacco has on the body or teeth.

Instruction (Methods)

1. Bring in food packages and demonstrate how to read the printed labels. Display a poster of the food pyramid and refer to as needed to reinforce nutritional information. Use an overhead transparency to explain the label reading concept as it pertains to food groups. Give examples of good and bad foods with emphasis on choosing healthy snacks.
2. Show projection slides of children with baby-bottle syndrome. Show the disease in its active state as well as cases where treatment has been done. List the types of liquid that cause baby-bottle syndrome in. English and in Spanish in on a flipchart. Emphasize prevention such as tooth brushing and choosing alternative liquids.
3. Illustrate the use of sealants with a flipchart. Also demonstrate on the typodont. Review the acid equation and decay, emphasizing prevention such as toothbrushing and good nutritional choices.
4. Use overhead transparencies to demonstrate the steps involved in treating a dental emergency. Show a dental emergency kit to students. Show a mouth guard to students.
5. Discuss tobacco and its effects on the body using a felt board with young man who is healthy, and the negative changes his body goes through as he begins to use tobacco. Show overhead transparencies of actual healthy and lungs with disease caused by tobacco use. Discuss smokeless tobacco and show pictures of it. Show alternative products to smokeless tobacco and allow students to try it (All Mint Chew by the Oregon Mint Snuff Co.). Display a poster of the different types and stages of oral cancer. Teach students where the most common places to find oral cancer are and how to examine themselves. Hand out mirrors for this exercise and demonstrate and give help where needed.

Lesson Plan continued

Visuals

1. A Poster of the food pyramid and overhead of a food label.
2. Food packages.
3. Slides depicting baby-bottle syndrome and its effects on the teeth.
4. Demonstration of sealants on the typodont and on a flip chart.
5. Overhead transparencies depicting the steps to take in a dental emergency.
6. An example of a mouth guard for students to touch and hold.
7. A dental emergency kit for students to examine.
8. Slides of diseased lungs due to tobacco use.
9. Felt board to illustrate the negative effects tobacco has on the body and teeth.
10. Flip chart of pictures of tobacco forms and types.
11. Examples of "All Mint Chew" for students to try.
12. Colored poster of the different stages and types of oral cancer.

Guided Practice Activities

1. Students will examine their mouths for signs of oral cancer.
2. Students will examine food labels.

Closure

1. Review topics briefly and ask students questions regarding the objectives.
2. Distribute pamphlets regarding the subjects covered.
3. Answer any questions the students may have.

Independent Practice

1. Encourage students to practice their new skills at home and to teach other family members.

Source: Susan Briones and Julie Herring

DENTAL HEALTH EDUCATION EVALUATION

STUDENT(S) _____   TEAM# _____   DATE _____

SCHOOL _____ TEACHER _____   GR _____

CRITERIA

5 EXCELLENT	Met all the outlined criteria
4 VERY GOOD	Met most of the outlined criteria
3 GOOD	Met some of the criteria outlined
2 FAIR	Some preparation exhibited, needs to review criteria
1 POOR	Little preparation exhibited, review criteria
0 Omitted	Information or material not covered

EVALUATION (Points possible)		COMMENTS	POINTS
ANTICIPATORY SET (5)	5 4 3 2 1 0		
OBJECTIVES (5 ¥ 2) (10)	5 4 3 2 1 0		
INSTRUCTIONS (50)			
Information	5 4 3 2 1 0		
Vocabulary	5 4 3 2 1 0		
Appropriate	5 4 3 2 1 0		
Audio-Visual	5 4 3 2 1 0		
Class Control	5 4 3 2 1 0		
Use of Time	5 4 3 2 1 0		
Level/Learning	5 4 3 2 1 0		
Creativity	5 4 3 2 1 0		
Enthusiasm	5 4 3 2 1 0		
Appearance (−5 no uniform)	5 4 3 2 1 0		
GUIDED PRACTICE (15 × 2) (30)			
Level/Learning	5 4 3 2 1 0		
Use of Time	5 4 3 2 1 0		
Provided help	5 4 3 2 1 0		
CLOSURE (5)			
Restate Objectives/ Check for Understanding	5 4 3 2 1 0		

ADDITIONAL COMMENTS

TOTAL POINTS (100)

CRIETERIA

ANTICIPATORY SET (5 points): Focus children, introductions, attention getter, setting the stage, standards, review last lesson, class control, costume, arrive on time, prepared, organized, ready to go.

OBJECTIVES (5 × 2=10 points): Clearly stated; behavior objectives, Maximum of 3, At grade level, Consistent with instructions.

INSTRUCTIONS (5 × 10=50 points): Accurate, clear, professional, proper Grammer, at level of understanding (watch "O.K." and "you guys"), follows scope and sequence, keeps on track of topic. *Visuals:* neat, clear, big enough, used well, cursive or printing at grade level. *Use of time:* uses the full half-hour, presentation does't drag on/rushed. *Level of learning:* meaningful lesson at classroom grade level (teach to the lowest level for a split class). *Creativity:* personal touch in applying scope & sequence. *Enthusiasm:* fake it if don't feel it—its contagious. *Appearance:* –5 no uniform (lab coat, name tag, flat shoes, and socks/nylons, no open toe sandals) or appropriate costume.

GUIDED PRACTICE; (15 × 2=30 points) *Appropriate:* follows instruction to the students level (comprehension, motor skills) demonstrates activity first. *Use of time:* well placed, enough time for activity. *Individual help:* critique students both positively and negatively, gives each student appropriate guidance as needed.

CLOSURE (5 points) Restate Objectives, summarize what was accomplished or ask students what they learned. Check for understanding. Time for Questions. Preview of next lesson. State what independent practice is needed (follow-up activity on their own).

ADDITIONAL COMMENTS (points added or deleted at instructor's discretion: May include comments about phrasing, articulation, voice quality, eye contact, and teamwork.

CHAPTER 16

The Oral Health of Older Americans

Currently, the trend is moving toward improvement of the oral health status among older adults (65 years and older). With this positive change, oral diseases and tooth loss can be minimized as teeth can be expected to last in good oral condition for a lifetime. Financing dental care continues to be a major problem for the older adult compared with other age groups. Few older adults are covered by private dental insurance, and it is left up to the state dental insurance programs to cover routine dental services. Therefore, dental care is sometimes unavailable for those living on a fixed income. However, the absence of proper oral healthcare can and often does lead to disastrous consequences for the older American. Additionally, as the older American population increases, there are challenges to providing care for the other adults, because the number of practicing dentists is declining. The dental care professionals licensed to provide care in special settings should be encouraged to provide as much care as possible to the older Americans. Continued improvement for the oral healthcare of this special population will be dependent on access to appropriate dental care and services.*

*Source: CDC Report. "The Oral Health of Older Americans." Aging Trends No. 3. www.cdc.gov/nchs/pressroom/01fact/olderame.htm.

When presenting information to older adults, the following facts should be well noted:

Facts

- Many older people are keeping their natural teeth. There is a big difference in income availability for oral healthcare at age 65 or older. Those in poverty are twice as likely to have lost all their teeth.
- Many older people take medications for chronic conditions that have side effects on oral health. The treatment for systemic diseases are sometimes complicated by oral bacterial infections.
- Oral health problems can cause pain when chewing, speaking, and swallowing, and the problems affects quality of life.
- One-third of older Americans (over 65 years) have untreated dental caries; slightly over 40 percent have periodontal disease.
- Only 22 percent of older Americans are covered by dental insurance.
- The average age for nursing home residents is now 81 years old. At current rates, there would be approximately three million residents in nursing homes in the year 2030, double the number in 2000.
- Oral cancer increases with age. Oral cancers result in 8,000 deaths each year; more of half of those deaths occur in those over 65 years of age.

Information presented should focus on the following areas of the state of oral health for older Americans:

- How oral health affects quality of life
- The link between oral care and systemic diseases
- Oral hygiene instructions, including adapted aids (toothbrush, flossing aides, etc.)
- Nutrition and dietary needs

- Oral pain
- Difficulty in eating
- Tooth loss (endentuluism)
- Effects, care, and cleaning of dental prostheses
- Problems with multiple medications
- Dental caries, periodontal diseases, and oral cancer
- Utilization of dental care services
- Dental insurance

Providing oral health information to the senior population can be a challenging and rewarding experience for both the dental health professional and the population of seniors that is served. Remember to keep the information simple. Two different examples of lesson plan outlines are provided. It is important to consider the amount of time and cognitive level of your audience. You may need to plan two or three short visits or presentations instead of one long presentation. Information can be added or deleted to the outline as needed. The use of visual prompts and aides, pictures, samples of products, etc. is helpful.

Lesson Plan

I. Review the importance of good oral health during all stages of life.
   A. A smile says a lot; providing information about health, hygiene, and self-esteem.
   B. Ability to eat depends on oral health; nutritional intake is important to prevent illness and maintain overall health.
   C. Dental diseases stress the entire body; pain, bacteria, infection may prolong illness and lead to more serious health problems.

II. Oral diseases and means of prevention
   A. Dental caries (tooth decay)
      1. Cause: plaque and bacteria combined with dietary carbohydrates (sugars)
      2 Preventive methods:
         a. Plaque removal: toothbrushing, dental floss, and other aids
         b. Fluoride applications: dentifrices, rinses, professional applications
         c. Proper nutrition: foods causing caries and alternative dietary choices
   B. Periodontitis (destruction of tissues supporting teeth)
      1. Causes: plaque and bacteria, stress (illness), poor oral hygiene
      2. Prevention: toothbrushing and flossing methods, rinses, early recognition and treatment

III. Looking into the mouth
   A. The resistant patient: needs reassurance, gentle touch, patience.
   B. Protecting the caretaker and the patient from injury and infection.
   C. Recognizing and describing abnormalities in the mouth.
      1. Typical changes caused by common medications
         a. aspirin burns, black hairy tongue, candida, xerostomia (dry mouth)
         b. common treatments for minor changes and irritations
      2. Lesions and growth occurring due to illness and irritations
      3. Refer for diagnosis and treatment
   D. Recognition and care of removable dental prosthesis (dentures and partial dentures)
      1. indications that removable teeth are present in the mouth
      2. importance of routine denture removal and cleaning
      3. methods of cleaning dentures
      4. technique to place identification on dentures

IV. Importance of oral health on socializing and self confidence
   A. Breath odor
      1. Rinses (without alcohol), chewing gum, dentrifrices
   B. Mobile teeth
      1. Denture adhesives
      2. Referral to dentist

Lesson Plan / IMPLEMENTING DENTAL HYGIENE SERVICES TO THE FRAIL ELDERLY: A DENTAL HYGIENIST PERSPECTIVE

I. Who are the "frail elderly"?
   A. The confined elderly, usually needing assistance with daily activities (ADL's), getting out of bed, walking, preparing and eating meals, bathing, personal hygiene, etc.
   B. Seniors who have some physical, mental, or financial constraint preventing them from traveling to the traditional dental office to care.
   C. The 1.3 million elder Americans, (65 years +) who reside in Skilled Nursing Facilities and 6.67 million who are homebound. Of those who are not institutionalized, 23% have some functional limitations with walking, getting outside, or personal hygiene. These limitations increases with age, and affect 60% of those 85 years and older.

II. What are the benefits of accessing dental hygiene services to this population?
   A. The goal of dental hygiene is to promote wellness through preventive methods. Preventive dental care, through patient assessment, treatment and education, addresses oral problems which increase with age.
      1. Aging often finds an increase in periodontitis including gingival recession. Both may result in an increased susceptibility to root caries.
      2. Pathology of the oral structures may lead to painful obstruction or infection. Both may reduce nutritional intake and challenge the health of the already compromised patient.
      3. Mobile teeth, large amounts of plaque, or materia alba pose the danger of becoming dislodged. Should the frail patient inadvertently aspirate any of these, life threatening pneumonia may result.
      4. Tooth loss in the elder patient often serves to confirm their fears of future loss of health, mobility, or independence. It also contributes to a lowered sense of self-esteem. These concerns lead to stress which may have a negative affect on the patient's overall health.

III. How does the dental hygienist address these needs?
   A. Prevent risk of medical emergencies, "Never treat a patient you don't know." Obtain thorough medical history.
      1. Consult with physician, nursing staff, family or conservator, patient and facility chart.
      2. Major areas of medical concern prior to hygiene treatment:
         a. Patients may require antibiotic premedication: orthopedic implants, cardiac valve disease, kidney dialysis, bone marrow transplants, chemotherapy.
         b. Patients may require postponement of anticoagulant meds: aspirin, coumadin.
         c. Patients may require special considerations when combative or prone to sudden movements: Alzheimer's disease, dementia, medication induced confusion.
         d. Patients may require a "best-time" scheduling:
            Arthritis patients move easier in the afternoon.
            Diabetics have more stamina after meals.
            Cardiac patients have more energy in the morning.
      3. Be prepared: vital signs, access to oxygen, emergency contact person or number, access to telephone.
   B. Communication leads to cooperation.
      1. Allow longer treatment time for the frail elderly; they move slower, often need a briefs rest during procedures.

Lesson Plan continued

2. Speak clearly, perhaps slower and louder. Provide written communications in large, dark print. Both will accommodate the patient with a reduced sense of hearing or sight.

3. Provide reassurance and encouragement before, during, and after treatment. Failing health has resulted in their being dependent, vulnerable, sometimes fearful and in pain. The institutionalized have the added stress of living in unfamiliar surroundings and dealing with strangers for every basic need.

C. Performing Oral Evaluation:

1. Use basic equipment for preliminary assessment. Keep it simple!
   a. less costly
   b. easier to transport, set up and take down
   c. less noise disturbance to patient and roommates

2. Conform to all aspects of Infection Control Program

3. Observe and record soft tissue abnormalities
   a. Xerostomia, Candidia, denture sore, oral cancer. . .
   b. Look for probable causes
   c. Treatments, preventive methods and products available
   d. Refer with report

4. Observe and record hard tissue abnormalities
   a. Caries, periodontitis
   b. Treatment methods
   c. Preventive methods and products available
   d. Refer with a report

5. Complete report forms for patient, referral to dentist, physician, facility and conservator or family caretaker.

D. Adapting services to patient's environment

1. Individualized treatment plan:
   a. Assess patient's health, tolerance, ability to cooperate, and functional .capability.
   b. Assess oral conditions from preliminary evaluation.

2. Additional supplies needed, (remember, keep it simple).
   a. Chart, including medical history and dental history
   b. Instruments: probe, explorer, curettes
   c. Patient products: dentifrice, toothbrushes, fluoride, mouth rinse
   d. Portable light, mouth props, disposable soft supplies
   e. Infection control barriers and materials

3. Patient positioning: use existing furniture
   a. Lounge chair, Geri chair
   b. Bed, sofa
   c. Wheel chair with head rest

E. Provide preventive education

1. Methods:
   a. Direct to patient or family caretaker
   b. In-service to facility staff

2. Plaque removal:
   a. Toothbrushes: manual, modified handles, power brushes
   b. Toothettes, finger cot. Avoid lemon glycerin swabs
   c. Dental floss, floss handles, power flossers
   d. Chemical assistance, monitor use: Rinses, dentifrice and topicals include: chlorhexidine, fluorides, desensitizing agents. Subgingival medicaments.

3. Care of Removal Prosthesis
   a. Identification marking
   b. Cleaning: brushes, methods, and effervescent solutions

Lesson Plan   continued

     c. Adhesives
     d. Refer

IV. Securing the referral dentist, mobile dentists
  A. Contact skilled nursing facility's consulting dentist
  B. Patient's private dentist
  C. Local dental association component, mobile dental services
  D. Dental schools and their programs
  E. Hygienist's employer

Source: Reprinted with permission from Charlotte Burruso, RDHAP of Visiting Denal Hygiene Service.

CHAPTER 17

Creating a Community Outreach Program

This section outlines an approach to preparing for a community outreach program and provides two sample programs. Dental health professionals can play an important role by participating in community outreach programs. Your participation will give the community an opportunity to explore various topics, careers, and issues surrounding dental health and education. Before volunteering or committing to participate in a community outreach program, you will need to get organized, target resources, secure educational materials, and implement and evaluate the program.

The following outline can provide a guideline to assist you as you prepare for your community outreach program.

Organization

To begin, you need to set an objective or goal for the program. Your planning should include the following components:

- Date and time
- Location (indoors or outdoors)
- Size of the group participating
- Equipment required (e.g., tables, chairs, blackboard, easel, audiovisual materials)
- Staff or volunteers needed (proportionate to group size, recruitment)
- In-service training requirements (preplanning, training to outline responsibilities, goals)
- Advertisement or publicity needed or provided if held in conjunction with another event (see handout at the end of this section.)

Resources

Identify various organizations and groups that you can contact for supplies and information. These might include:

- National, state, and local dental hygienists associations
- National, state, and local dental associations
- National, state, and local dental-assisting associations
- Dental hygiene, dental, and dental-assisting schools
- Community service groups
- Dental supply companies (Smart Practice, Henry Schuene, etc.)
- Local and county public health services
- Oral health professional sales distributors (Colgate, Procter & Gamble, Oral B, Johnson and Johnson, etc.)

Educational Materials

All materials developed for your program should:

- Be age-appropriate.
- Be multilingual, if appropriate for the community (e.g., in English and Spanish).

- Use universal signage (simple, clear symbols and drawings).
- Make use of visual aids (e.g., posters, models, toothbrushes, floss).
- Avoid copyright infringement.

Implementation

To carry out the program, you will need to provide for the following components:

- An outline of the program time schedule
- Advertisement/publicity
- Delegation of duties (stations, monitors, coordinators, etc.) during the program
- A list of supplies and other materials needed for the presentation
- Transportation and storage of supplies
- Setup
- Breakdown

Evaluation

After you have presented the program, you will want to evaluate the outcome to determine the success of your efforts:

- Whether or not you met your goals.
- How well participants have learned and retained the information presented.
- Whether a behavior change was exhibited.
- Whether a decrease in decay can be noted from previous examinations.

The remainder of this section consists of specific guidelines for presenting two types of outreach programs: a dental health fair and a parent education meeting. Remember, the most successful outcomes are always the result of advanced planning.

Community Outreach Program: Dental Health Fair*

PREPARATION

(one-hour in-service training)

Recruit volunteers from the dental professions to assist in the health fair (students in dental programs as well as members in the professional dental organizations within the community). Provide in-service training for the volunteers to familiarize them with the program and with their responsibilities. If workable, assign each new volunteer to a team in which one member has previous outreach experience and acts as a mentor to the rest of the team. Working in teams makes it easier to carry out activities at each station, especially with nonprofessional volunteers.

Children and parents visiting the dental health fair will walk through each station. Obtain samples of toothbrushes, floss, stickers, and other supplies several months in advance; these can then be given away to participants during the fair.

ANTICIPATORY PLANNING

(15 minutes)

- Review the instructions.
- Introduce presenters.
- Describe the goals of the program or the format of information to be covered at each station. If space or number of volunteers is limited, you can combine the stations to fit your needs.
- Review break and lunch times.
- Review the locations of emergency and restroom facilities.
- Have a resource and referral list available at Station 6 for parents.

INSTRUCTION/INFORMATION

(5–10 minutes per station)

In the following sample program, six stations are set up to discuss various topics relating to dental health. A dental screening is held at the last station, with a prize (sticker) given to children who complete the screening. Depending on the needs of your community, you may wish to add or substitute other topics.

Station	Topic
1.	Visiting the dentist; dental tools
2.	Diet and nutrition
3.	Decay process and fluoride
4.	Toothbrushing and flossing
5.	Oral injury prevention and the dental emergency
6.	Dental screening and prize

More than one topic may be included at each station.

Guided Practice Activities

(5–10 minutes per station)

STATION 1: VISITING THE DENTIST; DENTAL TOOLS (INSTRUMENTS)

Volunteers should explain what children would encounter on their first visit to the dentist. Among the areas to be covered at this station are:

- Introduction of the dentist, dental hygienist, and dental assistant
- What happens at the first visit
- The dental chart (a book about each child)
- Use of gloves, mask, eye protection, and gowns for infection control
- Radiographic pictures of the teeth and bone, panorex, bitewings, periapical, etc.

Volunteers can demonstrate typical instruments and explain terminology (refer to the glossary and the tooth talk terminology listing in the appendix for definitions of dental terminology). Among the items to be exhibited are:

- Patient hand mirror
- Mouth mirror
- Tooth counter (explorer)
- Straw or Mr. Slurpy (saliva ejector)
- Electric toothbrush (slow speed with disposable prophy angle)
- Large tooth model
- Tooth model with restorations (silver star, silver hat, sealants)

Visuals: A variety of infection control items used in the dental office, a tray of dental instruments (see preceding listing), and models.

STATION 2: DIET AND NUTRITION

Volunteers should be able to help children identify healthful foods and compare them with foods that are not healthful. Among the areas to be covered at this station are:

- The food pyramid and recommended servings
- Healthful foods (a basket of different foods can be provided; the children can then be asked to identify the healthful foods)

Visuals: Charts, posters, and handouts of the food pyramid and nutrition or diet-related facts. Consult your local dairy counsel for additional information.

STATION 3: THE DECAY PROCESS AND FLUORIDE

Volunteers should be able to teach about the decay process and describe how a cavity starts. They should explain how fluoride can strengthen teeth, making them more resistant to decay.

Decay Process

- Explain the decay process:

    Plaque + Sugar = Acid
    Acid + Healthy Tooth = Decay (cavities)

- Describe baby-bottle tooth decay. Explain how the decay process is accelerated when milk, formula, juice, or breast milk in a bottle is allowed to

remain in a baby's mouth. Explain when and how to wean infants off the bottle. Recommend dilution of juices and use of water in bottles.
- Using a large molar model, show how a small pit and fissure cavity can quickly enlarge into a big cavity that may cause discomfort.
- Using a model of two teeth, show how interproximal decay occurs.
- Show how disclosing tablets and solution can detect plaque on teeth.

Fluoride

- Describe how fluoride (a "tooth vitamin") can prevent tooth decay by making the tooth more resistant (strengthening the enamel). Explain that fluoride can be found in some foods and water. It may also be applied to teeth at the dentist's office.
- Highlight the different ways to receive fluoride: water, toothpaste, mouth rinse, tablets, and fluoride treatments at the dentist's office.

Visuals: Pictures of the decay process, decayed teeth, and baby-bottle tooth decay; disclosing tablets and solution; patient mirrors; various products containing fluoride. Pictures and videotapes may be available through the local dental society.

STATION 4: TOOTHBRUSHING AND FLOSSING

Volunteers should demonstrate how to choose a soft bristle toothbrush and the proper brushing technique. They should show examples of different types of floss and demonstrate proper flossing technique on a tooth model or in their mouth.

Toothbrushing

- Describe and provide examples of different types of toothbrushes (hard versus soft, small versus large, single and multiside).
- Emphasize the need for one toothbrush per person (do not share).
- Describe the qualities of a good toothbrush versus one that is worn out.
- Demonstrate the proper technique: brushing at a 45-degree angle to the gum line; using small, circular strokes angled into the gum line for the front and back of teeth; and using circular strokes on the chewing surfaces.
- Emphasize the need to brush the tongue after the teeth to remove bacteria on the tongue.

Flossing

- Demonstrate proper flossing technique, including the appropriate length of floss and the finger positioning.
- Emphasize the need for adult supervision.
- Demonstrate the use of a floss holder.
- Discuss and provide examples of types of floss available (children's flavor, mint fluoride, tape, waxed, unwaxed, and superfloss).

Visuals: A large tooth model, large toothbrush, pictures of proper toothbrushing and flossing technique, a variety of toothbrushes and floss. Hand out samples, if available, to participants.

STATION 5: ORAL INJURY PREVENTION AND THE DENTAL EMERGENCY

Volunteers should stress the importance of preventing oral injury by wearing a mouth guard for all contact sports and activities in which there is a risk of oral injury (baseball, basketball, football, soccer, in-line skating, skateboards, hockey, wrestling, etc.). They should also describe the types of mouth guards available and provide examples:

- *Boil and bite*: Purchased in a sporting goods store; softened in boiling water, then bitten down on to form an impression of the teeth; available in limited sizes and provides only limited coverage to the tops of teeth.
- *Custom-fit*: Made directly from a mold of the athlete's teeth; fits better, lasts longer (less distortion).

Dental Emergency Procedures

Volunteers should be able to describe the first aid that should be provided for the following common dental emergencies. Refer to the lesson on Dental Safety and Oral Injury Prevention in Section 2 for specific instructions to be given for each emergency.

- Bitten tongue
- Broken tooth
- Knocked-out tooth
- Objects wedged between the teeth
- Orthodontia problems
- Possible fractured jaw
- Toothache

Visuals: A variety of mouth guards and a large chart or poster describing dental emergency procedures. Handouts may be available through the local dental society.

STATION 6: DENTAL SCREENING AND PRIZE

A "look-and-see" screening for obvious dental problems will be done, and parents will be informed of any problems or needs that are identified. Complete screenings are not done during this session, and this visit does not take the place of a dental examination. Also available is the Early Childhood Caries (ECC) assessment screening form (CAT[C4]). Volunteers should be able to identify common dental problems and help reinforce good dental habits. Among the areas to be addressed at this station are:

- Ways to keep teeth happy and healthy, including regular visits to the dentist, healthful food choices, and good oral hygiene habits (brushing and flossing).
- Referral to the child's dentist if he or she needs immediate dental cares or give a referral list. (Orthodontics and routine dental care are not considered emergencies necessitating immediate care.)
- Caries-risk assessment screening form (example at the end of this section). Additional information can be downloaded from www.mchoral.org website.
  1. Clinicians should have access to historical information for nonclinical data elements.
  2. Assess all three components of caries.
  3. Note that when assessing information, use the highest risk category when a risk category exists.
  4. Additional information may be needed (X-rays, microbiologic testing, etc.).
  5. CAT can be used by dental and nondental personal.
  6. CAT does not render a diagnosis.
  7. CAT is intended to be used when clinical guidelines call for a caries-risk assessment.

Give a sticker (prize) to each child who participates so you know who has completed the "look-and-see" screening.

CLOSURE

(2–3 minutes at each station)

- Check participants' knowledge and understanding of the concepts presented.
- If time permits, address any other questions participants may have.

✔ Checklist

DENTAL HEALTH FAIR

- Copies of handouts.
- Provide in-service training.
- Obtain supplies.
- Assign specific stations and shifts.
- Reserve equipment (tables, VCR, monitor, videotapes, etc..)

Notify volunteers:

- Date and time
- What to bring
- What to wear
- Location (specific area)
- Coordinator's phone number(s)
- Other

Comments: _____

PATIENT INFORMATION ON TOOTH DECAY

How Tooth Decay Happens

Tooth decay is caused by certain type of bacteria (mutans streptococci and lactobacilli) that live in your mouth. When they attach themselves to the teeth and multiply in dental plaque, they can do damage. The bacteria feed on what you eat, especially sugars (including fruit sugars) and cooked starch (bread, potatoes, rice, pasta, etc.) Within about five minutes after you eat or drink, the bacteria begin producing acids as a byproduct of their digesting your food. Those acids can penetrate into the hard substance of the tooth and dissolve some of the minerals (calcium and phosphate). If the acid attacks are infrequent and of short duration, your saliva can help to repair the damage by neutralizing the acids and supplying minerals and fluoride that can replace those lost from the tooth. However, if your mouth is dry, you hove many of these bacteria, or you snack frequently; then the tooth mineral lost by attacks of acids is too great and cannot be repaired. This is the start of tooth decay and leads to cavities.

Methods of Controlling Tooth Decay

Diet: Reducing the number of sugary and starchy foods, snacks, drinks, or candies con help reduce the development of tooth decay. That does not mean you con never eat these types of foods, but you should limit their consumption particularly when eaten between main meals. A good rule is three meals per day and no more than three snacks per day.

Fluorides: Fluorides help make teeth more resistant to being dissolved by bacterial acids. Fluorides are available from a variety of sources such as drinking water, toothpaste, over-the-counter rinses, and products prescribed by your dentist such as brush-on gels used at home or gels and foams applied in the dental office. Daily use is very important to help protect against the acid attacks.

Plaque removal: Removing the plaque from your teeth on a daily basis is helpful in controlling tooth decay. Plaque can be difficult to remove from some parts of your mouth, especially between the teeth and in grooves on the biting surfaces of back teeth. If you have an appliance such as an orthodontic retainer or partial denture, remove it before brushing your teeth. Brush all surfaces of the appliance also.

Saliva: Saliva is critical for controlling tooth decay. It neutralizes acids and provides minerals and proteins that protect the teeth. If you cannot brush after a meal or snack, you can chew some sugar-free gum. This will stimulate the flow of saliva to help neutralize acids and bring lost minerals back to the teeth. Sugar-free candy or mints could also be used, but some of these contain acids themselves. These acids will not cause tooth decay, but they con slowly dissolve the enamel surface over time (a process called erosion). Some sugar-free gums are designed to help fight tooth decay and are particularly useful if you have a dry mouth (many medications can cause a dry mouth). Some gums contain baking soda, which neutralizes the acids produced by the bacteria in plaque. Gum that contains xylitol as its first listed ingredient is the gum of choice. If you have a dry mouth, you could also fill a drinking bottle with water and add a couple teaspoons of baking soda for each 8 ounces of water and swish with it frequently throughout the day. Toothpastes containing baking soda are also available from several companies.

Antibacterial mouthrinses: Rinses that your dentist can prescribe are able to reduce the number of bacteria that cause tooth decay and can be useful in patient at high risk for tooth decay.

Sealants: Sealants are plastic coatings bonded to the biting surfaces of back teeth to protect the deep grooves from decay. In some people, the grooves on the surfaces of the teeth ore too narrow and deep to clean with a toothbrush, so they may decay in spite of your best efforts. Sealants are on excellent preventive measure for children and young adults at risk for this type of decay.

CARIES RISK ASSESSMENT FORM FOR CHILDREN AGE 0 TO 5 YEARS

Instructions

1.   Respond to questions 1(a) through 1(j) and 2(a) through 2(f) with yes or no answers. You can make special notations such as the number of caries present, the severity of the lack of oral hygiene, the brand of fluorides used, the type of bottle contents used, the type of snacks eaten, or the names of medications/drugs that may be causing dry mouth.
2.   If the answer to any question in section 1 is yes for children old enough to spit (probably 4 or 5 years old), then a bacterial culture (**CRT bacteria test***) should be taken, as described below. For children not old enough to spit (3 years or younger), the bacterial levels of the parent/caregiver should be used as a rough estimate of the child's likely bacterial challenge. Saliva samples are taken from the mother or caregiver using the **CRT bacteria test*** (Vivadent)—see below. Children age 0 to 3 years are difficult to culture reliably in the fashion described below. However, an approximate indication for the child can be obtained by using a cotton swab to sample the surface of all teeth and gums in the mouth, thoroughly dispersing the sample in about 1–2 ml of water, and coating this on the test media strips as described below for saliva samples. Make an overall judgment as to whether the child is at high, medium, or low risk depending on the balance between the pathological factors (section 1) and the protective factors (section 2). Note! Determining the caries risk for an individual child requires evaluating the number and severity of the risk factors. Certainly, a child with caries presently or in the recent past is at high risk for future caries. A patient with low bacterial levels would need to have several other risk factors present to be considered at moderate risk. Some clinical judgment is needed while also considering the protective factors to determining the risk. Note! Children with developmental problems or low socioeconomic status are automatically at high risk. Place the completed form in the patient's chart.
3.   Provide the parent/caregiver with recommendations based on your clinical observations and the responses to the questions and discuss strategies for caries control and management. Give the parent/caregiver the sheet that explains how caries happens and the sheet with your recommendations. Copy the recommendations and place in the patient's chart.
4.   Inform the parent/caregiver of the results of any tests. Showing the parent the bacteria grown from their mouth (CRT test result*) con be a good motivator, so have the culture tube handy at the next visit (or schedule one for this purpose — the culture keeps satisfactorily for some weeks), or give/send them a picture. If the parent/caregiver has high cariogenic bacterial counts, then work with them and their own dentist to bring them to low caries risk and get their caries under control to eliminate this source of infection and re-infection for the child.
5.   After the parent/caregiver/child has been following your recommendations for three to six months, have them back to re-assess how well they are doing. Ask them if they are following your instructions—how often. If the bacterial levels were moderate or high initially, repeat the bacterial culture to see if bacterial levels hove been reduced. Make changes in your recommendations or reinforce protocol if results are not as good as desired or the patient is not compliant.

*Test procedures—Caries Bacteria Testing

***Bacterial testing:* CRT bacteria test:** In the United States, the currently available chairside test for cariogenic bacterial challenge is the Caries Risk Test (CRT) marketed by Vivadent (Amherst, NY). It is sufficiently sensitive to provide a level of low, medium, or high cariogenic bacterial challenge. It can also be used as a motivational tool for patient compliance with an antibacterial regimen. Other bacterial test kits will likely be available in the near future. The following is the procedure for administering the CRT test. Results are available after 48 hours.

The kit comes with two-sided selective media sticks that assess mutans streptococci on the blue side and lactobacilli on the green side.

(a)   Remove the selective media stick from the culture tube. Peel off the plastic sheet covering each side of the stick.
(b)   Pour the collected saliva over the media on each side until it is entirely wet.
(c)   Place one of the sodium bicarbonate tablets (included with the kit) in the bottom of the tube.
(d)   Replace the media stick in the culture tube, screw the lid on, and label the tube with the patient's name, registration number, and date. Place the tube in the incubator at 37 degrees Celsius for 48 hours. Incubators suitable for a dental office are also sold by the company.
(e)   Collect the tube after 48 hours and compare the densities of bacterial colonies with the pictures provided in the kit indicating relative bacterial levels. The dark blue agar is selective for mutans streptococci, and the light green agar is selective for lactobacilli. Record the level of bacterial challenge in the patient's chart as low, medium, or high.

CARIES RISK ASSESSMENT FORM FOR AGE 0 TO 5 YEARS

Instructions on reverse

Patient Name: _____ I.D. # _____ Age _____ Date _____

Initial/baseline exam date _____ Recall/POE date _____

Response to each question in sections 1, 2, and 3 with a check mark in the yes or no column			Notes
	Yes	No	
1. High Risk Factors**			
(a) Mother or primary caregiver has had active dental decay in the past 12 months			
(b) Child sleeps with a bottle, or nurses on demand			
(c) Bottle contains fluids other than milk or water			
(d) Obvious white spots, decalcifications, or obvious decay are present on the child's teeth			
(e) Recent dental restorations completed (less than two years)			
(f) Child's gums bleed easily and/or plague is obvious on the teeth			
(g) Frequent (greater than three times) between meal snacks of sugars/cooked starch			
(h) Appliances present, fixed or removable: e.g., space maintainers, obturators, etc.			
(i) Visually inadequate saliva flow (measuring saliva flow with young children is not possible)			
(j) Saliva-reducing factors are present, including:			
1. hyposalivatory medications (i.e., some for asthma or hyperactivity)			
2. medical (cancer treatment) or genetic factors			
(k) Child has developmental problems			
2. Protective Factors			
(a) Lives in fluoridated community			
(b) Mother or caregiver cleans child's teeth twice a day with fluoridated toothpaste (small amount)			Type _____
(c) Child has had a dental exam combined with oral hygiene instruction for the parent/caregiver			Type _____
(d) Salivary flow visually adequate			
(e) Mother or caregiver with moderate to high ms counts use xylitol gum or lozenges (4x per day)			Type _____ and % _____
(f) Mother/caregiver has no caries activity			

**If yes to any of 1(a)–(g), perform bacterial culture on mother or caregiver*	High Count* Date: ___	Moderate Count* Date: ___	Low Count* Date: ___	
(a) Mutans streptococci				(Place a check in the box below the count)
(b) Lactobacillus				(Place a check in the box below the count)
Child's caries risk status	**High**	**Moderate**	**Low**	**Circle High, Moderate or Low**
Recommendations given: yes _____ no: _____ Date given: _____ or Date follow up: _____				
* Indicates that rest descriptions for these procedures are on the following pages				

PARENT/CAREGIVER RECOMMENDATIONS FOR CONTROL OF DENTAL DECAY IN CHILDREN 0 TO 5 YEARS

Daily Oral Hygiene/Fluoride Treatment (These procedures reduce the bacteria in the mouth and provide a small amount of fluoride to guard against further tooth decay, as well as to repair early decayed areas)

_____   wipe baby's teeth with a small smear of fluoride toothpaste on a soft cloth (for babies)

_____   brush child's teeth with a fluoride-containing toothpaste (small smear or pea-sized amount) twice daily (for children old enough to have their teeth brushed by parent or caregiver)

_____   selective daily flossing of areas with early caries (while patches)

_____   other _____

Diet (The most important thing is to reduce the number of between-meal sweet snacks that contain carbohydrates, especially sugars. Substitution by snacks rich in protein, such as cheese, will also help)

_____   OK as is

_____   limit bottle/nursing (to avoid prolonged contact of milk with teeth)

_____   replace juice or sweet liquids in the bottle with water

_____   limit snacking (particularly sweets)

_____   replace high carbohydrate snacks with cheese and protein snacks

_____   other _____

Xylital (Xylitol is a sweetener that the bacteria cannot feed on. It limits the transfer of decay-causing bacteria from parent/caregiver to baby/toddler. Parents/caregiver with dental decay place their children at high risk. Parent/caregiver requires antibacterial treatment [see below]. Using xylitol-containing chewing gum or mints/lozenges is a way that parents/caregivers of high-risk children can reduce the transfer of decay-causing bacteria. This is most effective when used starting shortly after the child's birth.)

_____   Parents of children 3 and younger with high bacterial levels should use xylitol mints or xylitol gum 3–4 times daily

Antibacterial rinse (parents/caregivers)

_____   Parents/caregivers of children 3 years and younger with high bacterial levels should rinse with 10 ml of chlorhexidine gluconate 0.12% (***Periogard, Peridex, Oral Rx*** by prescription only). Rinse at bedtime 1 minute 1×/day for 2 weeks. Stop for two months. Repeat rinsing far 2 weeks

Practitioner signature _____   Date: _____

Parent/caregiver signature _____   Date: _____

CARIES RISK ASSESSMENT FORM FOR CHILDREN AGE 6 YEARS AND OLDER/ADULTS

Instructions

1. Respond to questions 1, 2, and 3 with yes or no answers. You can make special notations such as the number of caries present, the severity of the lack of oral hygiene, the brand of fluorides used, the type of snacks eaten, or the names of medications/drugs that are causing dry mouth.

2. If the answer is yes to question 1(a) or any two of questions 1(b) through 1(g), then a bacterial culture should be taken using the **CRT bacteria test*** (Vivadent)—see below. Make an overall judgment as to whether the patient is at high, medium, or low risk depending on the balance between the pathological factors (sections 1 and 2) and the protective factors (section 3). Note! Determining the caries risk for an individual requires evaluating the number and severity of the risk factors. Certainly, an individual with caries presently or in the recent past is at high risk for future caries. A patient with low bacterial levels would need to have several other risk factors present to be considered at moderate risk. Some clinical judgment is needed while also considering the protective factors to determining the risk. Note! Children with developmental problems or low socioeconomic status are automatically at high risk. Place the completed form in the patient chart.

3. Provide the patient with recommendations based on your clinical observations and the responses to the questions and discuss strategies for caries control and management. Give the patient the sheet that explains how caries happens and the sheet with your recommendations. Copy the recommendations for the patient chart.

4. Inform the patient of the results of any test results. Showing the patient the bacteria grown from their mouth (CRT test result*) can be a good motivator, so have the culture tube handy at the next visit (or schedule one for this purpose — the culture keeps satisfactorily for some weeks), or give/send them a picture.

5. After the patient has been following your recommendations for three to six months, have the patient back to re-assess how well he or she is doing. Ask if he or she is following your instructions—how often. If the bacterial levels were moderate or high initially, repeat the bacterial culture to see if bacterial levels have been reduced. Make changes in your recommendations or reinforce protocol if results are not as good as desired or the patient is not compliant.

*Test procedures—Saliva Flow Rate and Caries Bacteria Testing

*1. **Saliva flaw rate:** Have the patient chew a paraffin pellet (included with the CRT test—see below) for three to five minutes and spit all saliva generated into a cup. At the end of the three to five minutes, measure the amount of saliva (in milliliters) and divide that amount by lime to determine the ml/minute of stimulated salivary flow. A flow rate of 1 ml/min and above is considered normal. A level of 0.7 ml/min is low, and anything at 0.5 ml/min of less is dry, indicating a high-risk situation. Investigation of the reason for the low flow rate is an important step in the patient treatment.

*2. **Bacterial testing: CRT bacteria test:** In the United States, the currently available chairside test for cariogenic bacterial challenge is the Caries Risk Test (CRT) marketed by Vivadent (Amherst, NY). It is sufficiently sensitive to provide a level of low, medium, or high cariogenic bacterial challenge. It can also be used as a motivational tool for patient compliance with an antibacterial regimen. Other bacterial test kits will likely be available in the near future. The following is the procedure for administering the currently available CRT test. Results are available after 48 hours.

The kit comes with two-sided selective media sticks that assess mutans streptococci on the blue side and lactobacilli on the green side.

(a) Remove the selective media stick from the culture tube. Peel off the plastic cover sheet from each side of the stick.

(b) Pour the collected saliva over the media on each side until it is entirely wet.

(c) Place one of the sodium bicarbonate tablets (included with the kit) in the bottom of the tube.

(d) Replace the media stick in the culture tube, screw the lid on, and label the tube with the patient's name, registration number, and date. Place the tube in the incubator at 37 degrees Celsius for 48 hours. Incubators suitable for a dental office are also sold by the company.

(e) Collect the tube after 48 hours and compare the densities of bacterial colonies with the pictures provided in the kit indicating relative bacterial levels. The dark blue agar is selective for mutans streptococci and the light green agar is selective for lactobacilli. Record the level of bacterial challenge in the patient's chart as low, medium, or high.

CARIES RISK ASSESSMENT FORM FOR CHILDREN 6 YEARS AND OLDER/ADULTS
Instructions on reverse

Patient Name: _____ I.D. # _____ Age _____ Date _____
Initial/baseline exam date _____ Recall/POE date _____

Respond to each question in sections 1, 2, and 3 with a check mark in the yes or no column			Notes
	Yes	No	
1. High Risk Factors**			
(a) Visible cavitation (carious) or caries into dentin by radiograph			
(b) Caries restored in past three years			
(c) Readily visible heavy plaque on teeth			
(d) Frequent (greater than three times daily) between meal snacks of sugars/cooked starch			
(e) **Saliva-reducing factors:**			
1. Hyposalivatory medications			
2. Radiations to head and neck			
3. Systemic reasons, e.g. Sjögren's			
(f*) Visually inadequate saliva flow. (If yes, measure) less than 0.7 ml/min by test* low salivary flow or dry mouth			Amount: _____ ml/min
(g) Appliances present, fixed or removable, e.g. orthodontic brackets/bands/retainer or removable partial denture(s)			
2. Moderate Risk Factors			
(a) Exposed roofs			
(b) Deep pits & fissures/developmental defects			
(c) Interproximal enamel lesions/radiolucencies			
(d) Other white spot lesions or occlusol discoloration			
(e) Uses recreational drugs			
3. Protective Factors			
(a) Lives/works/school in fluoridated community			
(b) Uses fluoride toothpaste daily			Type _____
(c) Uses fluoride mouthwash/rise/gel daily			Type _____
(d*) Salivary flow visually adequates > 1 ml/min by test			
(e) Uses xylitol gum or mints 4 × day			Type _____ and % xylitol _____
(f) Mother/caregiver has no caries activity			Brand _____ Frequency _____

**If yes to 1(a) or any two of 1(b)–(g), perform bacterial culture*	High Count Date: ____	Moderate Count Date: ____	Low Count Date: ____	
(a) Mutans streptococci				(Place a check in the box below the count)
(b) Lactobacillus				(Place a check in the box below the count)
Caries risk overall (see over)	**High**	**Moderate**	**Low**	**Circle High, Moderate or Low**

Recommendations given: yes ____ no: ____ Date given: ____ or Date follow up: ____

* Indicates that test descriptions for these procedures are on the following pages

Source: © 2002 California Dental Association, California Dental Association hereby grants permission for the reproduction and use of this form by photocopy or other similar process, or by manual transcription, by health care practitioners, health care teachers, and their respective staff. All other rights are reserved.

PATIENT RECOMMENDATIONS FOR CONTROL OF DENTAL DECAY (AGES 6 AND OLDER/ADULT)

Daily Oral Hygiene (Aimed at reducing the overall bacteria in the mouth, especially at sites likely to decay. Choose the recommendations based on the danger sites and the condition of the mouth)

_____ brush twice daily (with fluoride toothpaste, all patients)   _____floss daily

_____ interproximal brush   _____ stimudents   _____toothpick   _____ superfloss

_____ other: _____

Diet (The most important thing is to reduce the number of between meal sweet snacks that contain carbohydrates, especially sugars. Substitution by snacks rich in protein, such as cheese will also help)

_____ OK as is _____ limit snacking _____ limit sodas_____other _____

Fluorides (All patients should use a fluoride toothpaste twice daily. Additional fluoride products should be added, depending on whether the risk level is medium or high. These fluoride products must be used daily to be effective)

_____fluoride-containing toothpaste 2×/day (all patients regardless of caries risk status)

_____fluoride rinse (0.05% NaF, **Act** or **Fluorigard**) 1× of 2×/day (use in addition to toothpaste. Patients at medium risk should rinse in the morning or last thing or night. For high risk patients use twice a day, once in the morning and once last thing at night. Continue long term with older patients or those who need or want extra protection)

_____**Prevident** "brush-on" nightly, **OR** ____ **gel** (**Prevident**) in custom tray 10 min/night (For high-risk patients, especially those with low saliva flow, or root caries, or active cavities. Continue until the risk status is lowered, then revert to fluoride as above)

_____fluoride lozenges (**Lozi-Flur or Fluar-a-day**) 1×/day (use for high-risk patients with with low saliva flow, such as radiation xerostomia. By dissolving in the mouth, these lozenges provide a concerntrated fluoride reservoir to protect against mineral loss and to enhance repair by remineralization. Dissolve slowly in mouth by holding the lozenge in a convenient place)

Sugar-free gum/mints (recommend for high risk patients, especially those with low saliva flow, and/or those who need to reduce in between meal snacking. The gums or mints that contain xylitol also have an antibacterial effect against the decay-causing bacteria. Preferably use a xylitol-containing gum.)

_____ Chew after meals when you cannot brush (xylitol preferred). _____ Use Xylitol mints 3–4 times daily.

Antibacterial rinse

_____Chlorhexidine gluconate, 0.12% (**Periogard, Peridex, Oral Rx**, available on prescription). Rinse with 10 ml at bedtime for 1 minute, 1×/day for 2 weeks. Stop for two months. Repeat rinsing for 2 weeks. Use fluoride rinse (see above) every day during the weeks in between.

For dry mouth

_____baking soda tooth paste with fluoride _____ baking soda gym—**Dental Care Gum** (Arm & Hammer. It contains baking soda and xylitol) or similar product. Chew frequently throughout the day.

_____rinse frequently with baking soda suspension during the day (fill sports water bottle with water and add 2 teaspoons of baking soda for each 8 oz. of water.)

Practitioner signature _____ Date: _____

Community Outreach Program: Parent Education Meeting

PREPARATION

(5 minutes before beginning lesson)

Display a variety of pacifiers; pictures of baby-bottle tooth decay; infant-sized and other toothbrushes; fluoride drops, tablets, and rinses; floss; models; flip charts; and a chart or handout of the food pyramid.

ANTICIPATORY PLANNING

(5 minutes)

- Review the previous presentation, if applicable.
- Introduce presenters.
- Describe the goal of the presentation: To educate parents about early childhood oral healthcare, prevention of dental problems, and feeding practices.

General Objectives

(2–3 minutes)

State specifically not more than three or four objectives appropriate for the audience that indicate what the majority of the attendees will be able to achieve by the completion of the program. Examples include:

- Describe the dental decay process.
- Identify the causes of baby-bottle tooth decay and how to prevent it.
- Recognize early infant oral habits and know how to modify or correct them.
- Utilize new information to make wise oral health decisions for children.

INSTRUCTION/INFORMATION

(40–60 minutes)

More than one topic may be included or combined with the guided practice segment (30 minutes).

- Discuss dental problems of early infancy, and dental disease among the school-age population.
- Present information on preventing baby-bottle tooth decay.
- Describe the causes of tooth decay and how it can be prevented.
- Discuss bedtime routines, use of pacifiers, and thumb sucking.
- Equate dental care with future smiles; discuss when to see a dentist, and how to find one.

Dental Problems of Early Infancy

Cavities and gum disease are the most common health problems in children. Cavities and gum disease are serious problems. Gum disease causes the gums to become red, sore, puffy, and to bleed easily. Cavities and gum diseases can cause pain and infection. Cavities in the baby teeth are just as serious as cavities in the permanent teeth. If baby teeth are lost too early, children do not learn to speak correctly, have difficulties with chewing, and the permanent teeth can come in crooked.

Ask parents if they have heard of baby-bottle tooth decay? Explain that it is a condition that occurs when a baby is put to bed with a bottle or is allowed to walk around with a bottle in the mouth that contains any liquid other than water. The pooling of sugary liquid in the baby's mouth causes severe cavities when left for long periods of time. The teeth can even rot down to the gums (*show visual*). This is a serious and painful problem. The best way to prevent this from happening is to hold a baby while feeding and avoid putting the baby to bed with a bottle. Explain that you will be teaching other ways to prevent baby-bottle tooth decay, such as toothbrushing, during this presentation.

Causes of Decay

Discuss what causes decay and how it can be prevented. Include the following topics:

- The decay process (Figure 4-1)
- Cleaning, brushing, and flossing needs of children from early infancy through the teenage years (Have samples of toothbrushes available to hand out to parents.)
- Benefits of fluoride
- Nutrition for dental health

Dental Disease Process

Explain that cavities and gum disease are both caused by germs growing on the teeth. When these germs group together, they are called plaque (*show visual*).

Proper Brushing

Describe the importance of brushing as a way to break up plaque germs and prevent gum disease and cavities, even baby-bottle tooth decay. Review proper brushing technique.

Pick a toothbrush with a soft bristle and a small head (*show examples appropriate for a child, teenager, and adult*). Demonstrate brushing on a Typodont (large tooth model), using small, circular strokes, and establishing a pattern. Pass out toothbrushes to those who would like them. Tell parents that before a baby has teeth, they should use a soft, clean cloth to clean the baby's gums. Explain that parents of toddlers should brush their teeth at least once a day to begin developing the habit of brushing. Caution that children aged 2 years and younger should not use toothpaste when brushing because they swallow it.

Finally, tell parents that they can help their child have healthier teeth by encouraging him or her to brush before school, after snacks, and before bed.

From Bottle to Cup: Preventing Baby-Bottle Tooth Decay

Prolonged bottle-feeding can lead to tooth decay. It can also promote overfeeding and prevent the baby from getting other needed nutrients from the diet.

By 7–9 months of age, a baby may be ready to learn to drink from a cup. At this age, a baby is developmentally able to sit up with support, grasp, and hold objects, and coordination is improving. This is the ideal time to introduce the cup. Some babies are suddenly ready to give up the bottle or to show an interest in learning. If this happens, parents should take advantage of the opportunity.

Parents should begin by replacing one bottle-feeding a day with a cup feeding. The meal at which the baby is most alert and rested is best or whenever he or she begins to show most interest. Tell parents not to expect the baby to know what to do at first. Parents should help by lifting the cup to the baby's mouth, tipping it to give the baby a small drink. In time, the baby will learn to do this by himself or herself. After a few days or weeks, parents can replace a second bottle-feeding with a cup feeding at a second meal or at snack time. They should continue to replace bottle feedings until the baby is no longer drinking from a bottle.

The baby may be fussy until he or she gets used to this new experience. Parents should be prepared for dribbling and spills. It may be messy at first, but emphasize that parents should take things slowly and be patient. Always reward the baby's success with kisses and cheerful words.

Emphasize that when choosing a cup, parents should choose one that is small and easy for the baby to lift and hold. The cup should be unbreakable. Some "training cups" have handles and a lid with a spout; others have a weighted bottom or a wide base to help prevent messy spills. Caution parents not to fill the cup to the top; they should pour only until it is half full.

Readiness to drink from a cup does not mean that the baby is ready to drink cow's milk. Parents should continue to use formula. Cow's milk should not be offered until the child's physician or other health care provider recommends it.

Finally, emphasize that it is best to introduce juices in a cup, not the bottle. Diluted juices can first be introduced at about 7 months of age. By 12–18 months, the baby should be drinking from a cup instead of a bottle. If parents have concerns related to weaning, they should discuss them with their pediatrician or other healthcare provider.

Bedtime Routines

Emphasize the importance of starting good oral health habits at an early age. Parents should establish a routine of brushing teeth before bed by the time a child reaches one $\frac{1}{2}$ year of age. Discuss the issues related to the use of pacifiers and thumb sucking.

Pacifiers

Discuss the variety of pacifiers available (orthodontic, etc.) and instructions for their use. Caution parents never to tie a pacifier around a baby's neck. Present the following guidelines for choosing a pacifier*:

- Look for a sturdy, one-piece construction, and a flexible, nontoxic material.
- Be sure the pacifier is too large to be swallowed.
- Make sure the shield or mouth guard portion cannot be separated from the nipple.
- Look for two ventilating holes.

Thumb-Sucking Habits

Advise parents that children should stop sucking their thumbs by the age of 2–3 years. The earlier thumb sucking is stopped, the better, and the less damage it will do. Preferably, thumb sucking will stop before the permanent teeth erupt (lower incisors). Caution parents that the longer the child maintains the habit, the greater the risk of improperly positioned teeth.

Discussion: Future Smiles

Discuss when to see a dentist and how to find one. Have available resources for care in the local area. Advise parents that the child's first appointment for a healthy dental checkup should occur between 6 months and one year of age to review fluoride content, vitamin supplements, baby bottle or breast feeding practice, etc.

Guided Practice Activities

(30 minutes)

This segment may be combined with the preceding instruction/information segment. Visual aids are included at the end of the lesson.

The "Give your Baby a Health Start" brochure may be passed out and discussed along with other health information or nutrition, etc. Areas that might be presented in an activity format include proper tooth-brushing and flossing technique, use of fluoride and sealants, and proper nutrition. This segment might include small group discussions or a question-and-answer session. Provide handouts for the dental health topics covered (see end of lesson and appendix).

TOPICS FOR PARENT TEACHING

Reinforce the following information for parents, using visual aids and demonstrating proper techniques. Provide written dental health information that parents can take with them and refer to later (see handouts at the end of this lesson).

Toothbrushing

Describe and provide examples of different types of toothbrushes (hard versus soft, small versus large, single and multiside). Emphasize the need for one toothbrush per person. Describe the qualities of a good toothbrush versus one that is worn out. Demonstrate the proper technique: brushing at a 45-degree angle to the gum line; using small, circular strokes angled into the gum line for the front and back of teeth; and using circular strokes on the chewing surfaces. Emphasize the need to brush the tongue after the teeth to remove bacteria on the tongue.

Flossing

Show various samples of floss. Explain that parents need to floss children's teeth to remove the plaque that builds up between the teeth where the toothbrush cannot reach. Younger children should floss with parent's guidance at least once a day. Floss holders may also be used. Demonstrate proper flossing, and have samples available for audience participation.

Fluoride

Explain that fluoride makes teeth stronger and helps prevent cavities. Hold up a glass of water as you explain that although certain foods contain fluoride (e.g., fish, green leafy vegetables, apples), the most cost-effective way to get fluoride is in water. When a community's water undergoes fluoridation, the right amount of fluoride is added to the water to prevent cavities. If the water is not fluoridated, parents should ask the child's doctor or dentist to prescribe fluoride for children between the ages of 3 and 16 years. Children may also receive fluoride treatments at the dentist's office. Explain that fluoride mouth rinses are recommended for children over the age of 6 years. Parents can also buy toothpaste with fluoride in it.

Sealants

Explain what sealants are and why they are used. Sealants are a plastic coating that is painted on the four permanent molars that appear when a child is about 6 or 7 years old, and the four molars that emerge when a child is about 12 or 13 years old. They help to prevent cavities in the tops of the teeth. Explain that sealants are usually applied at a dentist's office. The process does not hurt at all. The coating is usually painted on the tooth and is given time to dry.

Nutrition

Present a visual depiction of the food pyramid. Explain that for healthy bodies and healthy teeth, we need to eat foods from all the groups shown on the pyramid.

Reinforce the idea that although a balanced diet is important in preventing cavities, tooth decay is also the result of what, when, and how often children eat. Explain that frequent snacking leaves food on the teeth longer and thus is more apt to promote the decay process. For this reason, sugars and starches are best reserved for mealtime, when increased saliva production helps neutralize the acids produced by oral bacteria.

Discuss how research has shown that certain foods have anticavity power, that is, they reduce the acid exposure to the teeth. These foods are considered more dentally sound because they fight plaque and neutralize the bacteria that cause decay. They include:

- Cheese (e.g., Jack, cheddar, Swiss)
- Raw fruits and vegetables
- Peanuts and cashews

CLOSURE

(2–3 minutes, 5–10 minutes for questions)

- Restate the objectives in question form.
- Check attendees' knowledge and understanding of the concepts presented.
- If time permits, address any other questions attendees may have.

Lesson Plan: COMMUNITY OUTREACH PROGRAM: PARENT EDUCATION MEETING

DATE _____ LOCATION_____

TIME (60–90 MINUTES) _____ CONTACT PERSON _____

PRESENTER(S)_____

Preparation in Classroom _____
_____
_____
_____
_____
_____

Anticipatory Planning _____
_____
_____
_____
_____
_____

Review of Previous Objectives: _____
_____
_____
_____
_____
_____

Three Specific Objectives:

1. _____
_____

2. _____
_____

3. _____
_____

Lesson Plan continued

Information to be Presented Will Include:

(Topics) _____

_____

_____

_____

_____

_____

(Methods) _____

_____

_____

_____

_____

_____

(Lecture, Demonstration, Visual aids, Group discussion) _____

_____

_____

_____

_____

_____

Guided Practice Activities _____

_____

_____

_____

_____

_____

Closure _____

_____

_____

_____

_____

_____

_____

Dental Health Fact Sheet

FOOD FOR DENTAL HEALTH

Sugary foods are harmful to the teeth. It is important to limit the daily intake of sweet foods. Here are some ideas for good snack foods:

Nuts	Fresh fruits and vegetables
Sunflower seeds	Unsweetened juices
Popcorn	Sugarless gum, candy, soft drinks
Pretzels	Luncheon meats, beef jerky
Cheese	Leftover roast beef or chicken

Your Dentist

This school program does *not* take the place of regular dental checkups. It is important for your child to visit a dentist at least two times a year for checkups and/or dental repairs.

How You can Help at Home

- Encourage your child to practice brushing and flossing at home everyday (particularly before bedtime at night). It is important for you to watch the flossing and help your child so the gums will not be injured.
- As your child learns to do a good job of tooth cleaning, ask him or her to teach the rest of the family.

Children learn best by watching adults. Be a good role model; practice proper dental hygiene everyday!

Healthy teeth and gums . . . they can last a lifetime!

Dental Health Fact Sheet

Dental disease can be prevented and your teeth *can* last a lifetime. Unfortunately, 8 out of 10 children have dental disease by the age of 9 years. More than 95 percent of adult Americans have dental disease, and 20 million Americans have lost all their teeth. All this can be prevented if everyone would learn and practice personal dental care!

Your child's class is taking part in a "Smile in Style" Dental Disease Prevention Program. Students will learn ways of caring for their teeth and gums. Dental disease can be controlled if we practice daily care by brushing and flossing. To reinforce good dental habits, tooth cleaning and choosing good, nutritious foods must be done at home everyday in order to get the best results. Your participation is important.

Your Child Is Learning

- Teeth are important for eating, talking, happy smiles, and good health.
- There are two major dental diseases caused by germs living on and around the teeth: Tooth decay (cavities) and gum disease (gingivitis or pyorrhea).
- Some of the germs live in a sticky, hard-to-see film called plaque. Plaque forms on teeth everyday.
- Plaque Germs + Sugar (in *all* foods) + Acid = Tooth Decay
- Germ Plaque + Toxins (plaque waste product) = Gum Disease
- Dental disease *can* be prevented. Help keep your teeth and gums healthy!
- Clean teeth daily with a toothbrush and dental floss.
- Eat fewer sugary foods, especially between meals.
- Help teeth fight decay by using some form of fluoride (fluoride toothpaste, fluoride tablets, topical applications by a dentist, or a weekly fluoride mouth rinse).

Information You Should Know

Always giving your child a bottle of milk or sweetened drink to take to bed can lead to serious tooth decay, known as baby-bottle tooth decay. When a baby falls asleep with a bottle in his or her mouth, the milk, or sweet liquid stays around the teeth. Germs and sugar create acid, which causes teeth to decay. Young children who walk around all day with a bottle in their mouth may also get many cavities for the same reason.

Your Child Is Learning to Use these Things to Clean His or Her Teeth

Toothbrush

A small toothbrush with soft, rounded bristles should be used to remove germ-filled plaque from teeth and gums.

- *Brush biting surfaces:* On the tops of teeth where you chew, the bristles should be pointed toward the grooves and moved gently back and forth.
- *Vibrate gently on both sides:* On cheek side and tongue side, bristles should be pointed toward the gum line and rocked gently in a short, wiggly motion. Children are cautioned not to scrub vigorously back and forth on these surfaces, as it can hurt the gums.

Dental Floss

Floss should be used to clean between the teeth where the toothbrush cannot reach. Most serious tooth decay and gum disease starts in these spaces. Each space has two tooth walls that must be cleaned. Start where the two teeth touch and clean all the way into the gum line space.

- Hold a 12–18-inch piece of floss by wrapping the ends around your middle fingers. Guide the floss between your teeth by holding it with your thumbs and first fingers.
- Curve the floss around one tooth and move it up and down gently several times, then curve it around the other tooth and move up and down before going on to the next space.

Fluoride Rinse and Fluoride Tablet Programs

Both programs are used in the classroom by parental permission only.

- *Fluoride rinse program:* The fluoride rinse is a solution that is used once a week. It is swished around in the mouth for a minute, and then it is spit out into a cup.
- *Fluoride tablet program:* The fluoride tablet is used daily after brushing. The tablet should be chewed for 30 seconds, swished for 30 seconds, and then swallowed.

Fluoride in either form strengthens teeth, providing protection against the cavity-causing agent, plaque.

*Source: Dental health fair information courtesy of U.O.P. Janet Chan Fricke.
**Source: Guidelines for safe use of pacifiers by Dr. Arthur J. Nowak.

Oral Health Information Outline

Plaque	Toothbrush	Flossing	Fluoride	Nutrition	Oral Cancer	Prosthetics	Oral Piercing	Whitening
Bacteria	Manual	Types of floss	Over the counter	Dietary guidelines	Early warning signs	Denture/Partials	Effects on the area	Home/office products
Disease process	Power	Hand flossing	RS	Cariogenic foods	Examination procedures	Cleaning	Proper care and cleaning of appliance	Sensitivity
Tarter	Size, handle	Floss holders	Tooth paste	Food intake	High Risk areas	Deposits	Signs and symptoms of problems	
Calculus	Problem areas	Bridge threaders	ADA seal	Diets effect on gingival tissue	Tobacco products	Types of cleaners		
Tooth loss	Abrasion		Rinse			Labeling		
Bone loss	TB		Tablet					
Bad breath	Procedures		Water					
	Bristles		Foods with fluride					
	Tongue							
	Brushing							
	Frequency							

Use Fact Sheets to Supplement Information

Sealants	Early Childhood Caries	Dental Office Visit	Highlights
What they are	Baby bottle tooth decay prevention	How often should you visit the dental office?	1. Bring samples of products discussed (toothbrushes, floss, etc.)
Recommendation for use	Early screening assessment	Professional Careers	2. Allow time for questions and answers
How long do they last			3. Do not cover too much information in one visit
			4. Keep it simple and have fun!
			5. Survey participants ahead of time to address their needs
			6. Survey participants after presentation to see if their needs were met

GUIDELINES FOR ORAL HEALTH PRESENTATION

The following is a list of topics to be presented. Fill in the time line as appropriate for your scheduled presentation. You may use all or some of the topics listed based on the amount of time and number of times you can present information. Supplement your information with the fact sheets on various dental care topics found in the appendix section.

Topic	Amount Of Time

Plaque Control _____
   a. Health Dentition
   b. Etiology of plaque and calculus development
   c. Caries development
   d. Gingivitis and periodontal disease
   e. Disclosing solutions
   f. Bad breath/mal odor

Toothbrushing _____
   a. Manual
   b. Powder
   c. Types of toothbrushes
   d. Storage

Flossing _____
   a. Flossing techniques
   b. Types of floss
   c. Floss holders

Care of prostheses _____
   a. fixed
   b. removal

Fluoride _____
   a. mouthrinses and gels
   b. fluoride dentifrices

Toothpaste (dentifrices) _____

Auxillary oral hygiene aids
   a. proxy brush, rubber tip, perio aid, tongue scrapper

Antimicrobial products _____

Whitening products _____

Nutrition and its relationship to good oral hygiene _____

Tobacco Education _____

Give Your Baby a Healthy Start

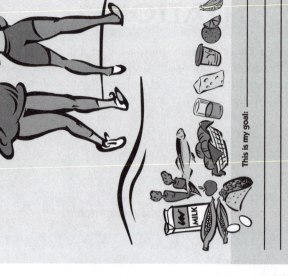

This is my goal: _____

How much weight will I gain while I'm pregnant?

Most women should gain between 25 and 35 pounds (11–16 kilograms). You will need to gain a little more if you were thin when you got pregnant. You should gain a little less if you were heavy when you got pregnant.

Your baby will probably weigh between 6 and 9 pounds. And you will need to gain some extra weight to help your baby grow.

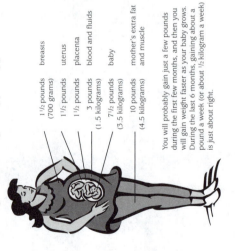

1½ pounds (700 grams)	breasts
1½ pounds	uterus
1½ pounds	placenta
5 pounds (1.5 kilograms)	blood and fluids
7½ pounds (3.5 kilograms)	baby
10 pounds (4.5 kilograms)	mother's extra fat and muscle

You will probably gain just a few pounds during the first few months, and then you will gain weight faster as your baby grows. During the last 6 months, gaining about a pound a week (or about ½ kilogram a week) is just about right.

Can I smoke or drink while I'm pregnant?

Cigarettes, drugs and alcohol (even beer or wine) could hurt your baby. If you need help to stop smoking, drinking or using drugs, ask your doctor or WIC staff for help.

Ask your doctor if it is OK before you take any pills, even aspirin.

Can I exercise while I'm pregnant?

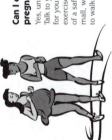

Yes, unless your doctor says not to. Talk to your doctor about what is best for you. Walking or other gentle exercise helps you feel good. Think of a safe place, maybe a park or a mall, where you can take walks. Try to walk every day.

Who can I talk with if I have questions about my pregnancy?

Keep your appointments at your doctor's office. The people there will answer your questions. They will also listen to your baby's heartbeat and make sure you and your baby are fine. The WIC staff are also there to answer your questions.

I think I'd like to breastfeed my baby, but I don't know much about it.

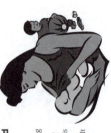

Find out more about breastfeeding now, while you are still pregnant. The WIC staff can give you lots of information and help! Breastmilk is best for your baby. Breastfeeding will help keep your baby healthy. It can even help you get your body back in shape!

Having a healthy baby sounds like a lot of work. How can I do it all?

Do what you can. Make changes a little at a time. You CAN make a difference in how your baby grows. And, take good care of yourself. Babies need strong, healthy moms!

Washington State Department of **Health**

DOH Pub 961-191 8/2004

Adapted from California State Department of Health, WIC Supplemental Nutrition Branch. Printed by Washington State Department of Health WIC Program. WIC is an equal opportunity program. For persons with disabilities this document is available on request in other formats. To submit a request please call 1-800-525-0127 (TDD/TTY 1-800-833-6388).

One Serving Is About....

6 to 11 servings each day

Breads, Grains, Cereals

Bread slice, tortilla, roll, muffin, pancake, bagel	1
Dry cereal	¾ cup or 180 mL
Noodles, rice, cooked cereal	½ cup or 120 mL
Crackers	8

Eat some whole grain foods every day.

3 to 5 servings each day

Vegetables

Cooked	½ cup or 120 mL
Raw	1 cup or 235 mL

Eat a dark green or yellow vegetable every day, like carrots, broccoli, spinach, greens, sweet potato, or squash.

2 to 4 servings each day

Fruits

Fresh	1 medium
Canned or frozen	½ cup or 120 mL
Juice	6 ounces or 180 mL

Eat a good vitamin C fruit every day, like orange, strawberries, melon, mango, papaya, or WIC juices.

3 to 4 servings each day

Milk Products

Milk	8 ounces or 240 mL
Cheese	1½ ounces or 45 g
Cottage cheese	2 cups or 475 mL
Yogurt, pudding or custard made with milk	1 cup or 235 mL
Frozen yogurt, ice cream	1½ cups or 355 mL

Choose mostly lowfat or fat free milk products.

2 to 3 servings each day

Protein Foods
Animal Protein

Meat, chicken, turkey, fish	2–3 ounces or 60–90 g
Eggs	2–3

Vegetable Protein

Cooked dry beans, peas, lentils	1 cup or 235 mL
Peanut butter	4 tablespoons or 60mL
Tofu	½ cup or 120 mL

Eat some vegetable protein foods every day!

Fats, Oils, and Sweets

It is OK to eat these foods once in a while.

Give your baby a healthy start!

So, you are going to have a baby!

Good for you! There are lots of things you can do to make this a happy, healthy time.

Does it matter what I eat while I'm pregnant?

Yes! Eating well while you are pregnant will help keep you strong and build a healthy baby.

This food guide will help you plan healthy meals and snacks. Try to eat more foods from the bottom of the pyramid and only a little bit from the top!

Drink lots of liquids, especially water. Drink milk and 100% fruit juices too. All milk has the same vitamins and minerals, whether it is nonfat, 2% or whole milk. Ask the WIC staff for more ideas.

One cup of coffee, tea, or soda a day seems to be fine.

Did your doctor tell you to take prenatal vitamins? These are important — don't forget them.

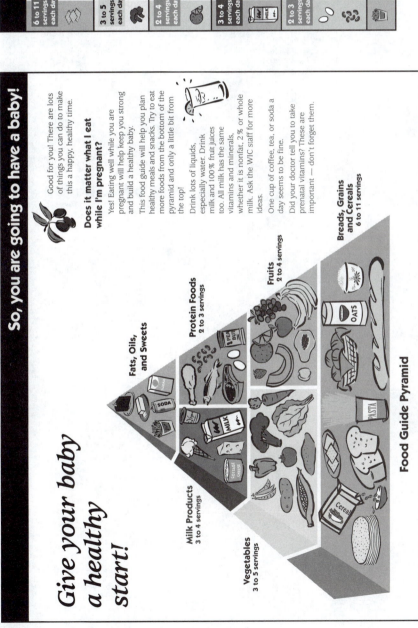

Fats, Oils, and Sweets

Protein Foods
2 to 3 servings

Fruits
2 to 4 servings

Milk Products
3 to 4 servings

Vegetables
3 to 5 servings

Breads, Grains and Cereals
6 to 11 servings

Food Guide Pyramid

Appendix: Additional Resources

The seven dental health fact sheets included in this appendix were developed by the Arizona Department of Oral Health, Kristy Menage Bernie, and other sources. Fact sheets are included on the following topics:

- Baby Bottle Tooth Decay (also known as Early Childhood Caries (ECC))
- Brushing Your Teeth
- Caring For Your Dentures
- Dental Sealants
- Flossing Your Teeth
- Fluoride to Prevent Tooth Decay
- Oral Cancer
- Oral Injury Prevention-Mouthguards
- Quiting Spit Tobacco
- Periodontal Disease
- Tobacco Facts
- Fresh Breath Assurance
- Putting Your Best Smile Forward: Tooth Whitening Options
- Fluoride Products for Home Use

Some fact sheets are presented first in English and then in Spanish translation. This information may be copied and distributed as needed. Also included in the appendix are a vocabulary list of dental terminology with definitions modified for children, a fluoride guidel update and a resource guide to additional supplies and contacts for more dental health related information.

You may also want to consult

- Oral piercing: www.aap.org (Oral Piercing Risk and Safety measures)
- ADHA.org (consumer and professional fact sheets on Oral Health)
- ADA.org (consumer and professional fact sheets on Oral Health)
- CDHA.org (consumer and professional fact sheets on Oral Health)

For more information.

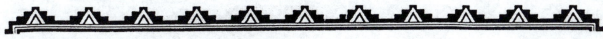

Oral Health Fact Sheet

Baby Bottle Tooth Decay

What is Baby Bottle Tooth Decay?

When an infant or small child develops several cavities, usually on the top front teeth, this is called Baby Bottle Tooth Decay. These cavities may look like dark pits, holes or broken teeth and may cause toothaches and make it hard for the child to eat.

What Causes Baby Bottle Tooth Decay?

It happens when liquids that contain sugar are left in a baby's mouth for long or frequent periods of time. Even breast milk and formula contain sugar.

How Can You Protect Your Child's Teeth?

Your child should **NOT**:

- go to bed with a bottle filled with milk, formula, juices or sweetened drinks
- sleep at night at the breast
- drink from a bottle throughout the day
- use a pacifier if it is dipped in honey, syrup or anything sweet, such as jello water, soda pop, fruit juices, kool-aid, sugar water, milk or formula

Your child **SHOULD**:

- start drinking from a cup at six months of age and be weaned from their bottle by one year of age
- go to bed <u>without</u> a bottle - if your child must have a bottle to sleep, fill it with plain water - you may need to mix the drink in the bottle with water, a little more water each night, until your child is drinking plain water
- have their teeth cleaned after each feeding with a clean washcloth, gauze pad, or a soft infant toothbrush - it is very important to clean your baby's teeth before bedtime!

Are Baby Teeth Important?

Baby teeth are important for chewing of food, proper speech, and they also give your child a nice appearance and good self image. If they are lost too early, the permanent teeth can come in crowded or out of line. Be sure your child visits a dentist before two years of age - your early efforts will be the key to your child's future dental health!

If you need this publication in alternate format, please contact us with your needs at
1-800-367-8939 (State TDD/TTY Relay) or 602-542-1866.

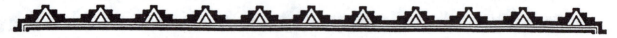

Oral Health
Fact Sheet

Daño De Dientes Por La Tetera

¿Qué es Daño De Dientes Por La Tetera?

Cuando el bebé o niño tiene varios caries en los dientes de enfrente y arriba se le nombra Daño de Dientes por la Tetera. Estas caries parecen hoyos negros o dientes rotos. Pueden causar dolor y dificultades en comer.

¿Qué Causa Daño De Dientes Por La Tetera?

Resulta cuando se le da al niño con frequencia líquados azucarados que se acumulen en la boca durante largos períodos de tiempo. La leche del pecho y la fórmula contiene azúcar también.

¿Cómo Puede Proteger Los Dientes De Su Bebé?

Su niño **NO DEBE**:
- acostar con una tetera llena de leche, fórmula, o bebida endulzada
- dormir toda la noche mamando el pecho
- tomar tetera durante todo el día
- usar un chupón cubierto con azúcar, miel, or otra cosa dulce como sodas y jugos.

Su niño **DEBE**:
- tomar de la taza a los seis meses y dejar la tetera a un año
- acostar <u>sin</u> la tetera - si su niño tiene que estar tomando para poder dormir, llénesela con agua. Si no la quiere con sólo agua, póngale leche pero poca a poco disuélvasela con más agua hasta que sea sólo agua.
- limpiar los dientes y la encía con una toalla limpia o un cepillo de dientes pequeño y suave. ¡Es muy importante limpiar los dientes del niño antes de acostar!

¿Son Importantes Los Dientes De Leche?

Los niños necesitan dientes fuertes y saludables para masticar sus alimentos, hablar y tener una sonrisa atractiva. Si pierde prematuramente un diente de leche, es posible que no le quepan los permanentes y pueden salirle torcidos o amontonados. Empieze las visitas al dentista antes de tiene dos años. ¡Sus esfuerzos hoy seran la llave a la salud dental en el futuro de su niño!

Si necesita esta publicación en diferente formato, llame al numero
1-800-367-8939 (State TDD/TTY Relay) or 602-542-1866.

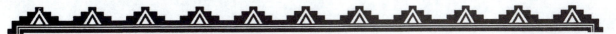

Oral Health Fact Sheet

Brushing Your Teeth

- Your teeth are meant to last a lifetime! Tooth decay or cavities, and periodontal disease, also known as gum disease, can be avoided or reduced by the daily removal of plaque.

- Plaque is made up of germs that live on your teeth, all the time. It is important to remove this plaque daily to prevent these germs from making acid and other products that can cause cavities and harm your gums and the bone around your teeth.

- If you spend less than three minutes brushing your teeth, probably all the plaque is <u>not</u> being removed. Also, a toothbrush with worn-out bristles cannot clean your teeth properly. Try to replace your toothbrush at least every three to four months.

- A dental home care plan should include:
    - daily toothbrushing with a **<u>soft</u>** toothbrush that is not worn out or frayed
    - using dental floss daily to clean the areas your toothbrush cannot reach that are
        between your teeth and under the gumline
    - using a toothpaste or mouthrinse with fluoride
    - eating balanced meals and limiting foods high in sugar

- To brush away the plaque on your teeth, follow these steps:

«Start by brushing the sides of your teeth that touch your cheek. Angle your toothbrush so it is up against your teeth and gums and jiggle the toothbrush back and forth in small strokes. Do only a few teeth at a time, and do it several times in each spot.

When you have completed the cheek side of your » top and bottom teeth, brush the side that faces your tongue on the top and bottom teeth in the same way.

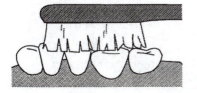

Brush the flat, chewing surfaces of your top and bottom teeth. These surfaces have many deep grooves where germs can "hide out." Brush your tongue when you finish brushing your teeth to help your mouth feel fresher. To maintain the health of your teeth and gums, clean in between your teeth with dental floss after toothbrushing.

If you need this publication in alternate format, please contact us with your needs at
1-800-367-8939 (State TDD/TTY Relay) or 602-542-1866.

Oral Health
Fact Sheet

Cepillandose Los Dientes

- ¡Sus dientes deben durar toda la vida! Las caries y enfermedad periodontal se pueden evitar o eliminar con quitar la placa diariamente.

- La placa contiene germenes que viven en los dientes constantemente. Es muy importante quitar la placa diario para prevenir que las germenes hagan ácidos y productos que causan caries y dañan las encías y el soporto de huesos del diente.

- Si no dura más de tres minutos cepillandose, **no** se está quitando la placa. Un cepillo con las cerdas gastadas no puede limpiar adecuadamente. Reponga el cepillo cada 3 o 4 meses.

- El cuidado dental en casa debe incluyir:
    - cepillar diario con cepillo suave y que no esté gastado
    - usar el hilo dental diario entre los dientes y debajo de las encías
    - usar pasta o enjuagues con fluoruro
    - comer buenos alimentos y limitar las comidas con mucho azúcar

- Para quitar la placa, haga lo siguiente:

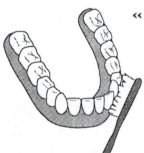

‹‹ Comience con el lado del diente que toca el cachete. Mueva en ángulo que quede hacia el diente y la encía y cepille hacia adelante y atrás en movimientos cortos. Haga unos cuantos dientes a la vez y quedece en lugar un tiempo.

Cuando termine el lado del cachete, cepille el ›› lado hacia la lengua arriba y abajo en el mismo modo.

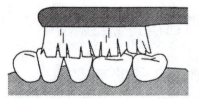

Cepille lo plano del diente arriba y abajo. Estos lugares tienen ranuras donde esconden los germenes.

Después de cepillar los dientes, cepille la lengua para sentirse mas fresco. Use el hilo dental después de cepillar.

Si necesita esta publicación en diferente formato, llame al numero
1-800-367-8939 (State TDD/TTY Relay) or 602-542-1866.

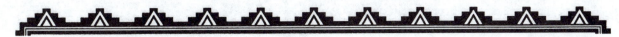

Oral Health Fact Sheet

Caring for Your Dentures

It is important to clean your mouth and denture daily so your mouth will stay healthy. It isn't enough to soak your dentures in water or a denture cleaner. They must be brushed with a soft toothbrush, or a toothbrush made especially for dentures.

Be sure to brush and massage your gums daily with a soft toothbrush, and brush any remaining natural teeth you may have.

- <u>Do not</u> clean a denture with boiling water.
- Clean all the surfaces of your denture, both inside and outside, with a denture brush and denture cleaner that you can buy at a drug store. <u>Do not</u> use an abrasive cleaning powder like Ajax or Comet.
- When cleaning a denture, hold it over a bowl of water between your thumb and forefinger. If it slips out of your hand, it will land in the water and not break.
- If a denture smells, it can be soaked in a solution of 1 teaspoon of bleach (Clorox) in one cup of water. Soak the denture for 30 minutes. Rinse the denture well before putting it back in your mouth.
- Take your denture out of your mouth for at least 8 hours every day. When it is out of your mouth, keep the denture in a bowl of water or diluted mouthwash.
- <u>Do not</u> try to adjust a denture with sandpaper or files - they will ruin the denture. <u>Do not</u> use denture liners or denture adhesives.

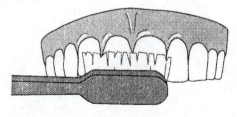 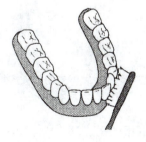

<u>Go To The Dentist for the Following</u>:
- Your regular fitting appointments after you get a denture
- When you have mouth sores that last for more than 1 week
- When your dentures become loose in your mouth
- One time a year to check the health of your mouth and the fit of your denture

If you need this publication in alternate format, please contact us with your needs at
1-800-367-8939 (State TDD/TTY Relay) or 602-542-1866.

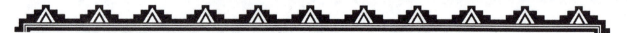

Oral Health
Fact Sheet

Cuidado de las Dentaduras Postizas

Es importante limpiarse la boca y la dentadura postiza diariamente para la buena salud oral. No es suficiente sólo remojar en agua o limpiador de dentaduras. Debe limpiar con una cepillo suave o con un cepillo especialmente para las dentaduras postizas.

Esté seguro de cepillar y masajear las encías diariamente con un cepillo suave. Cepille cualquier dientes naturales que todavía le quedan.

- **No debe** hervir la dentadura en agua caliente.
- Limpie todos superficies de la dentadura, por dentro y afuera, con cepillo y limpiador de dentaduras postizas. **No use** limpiadores abrasivos como Ajax o Comet.
- Cuando limpie la dentadura, sostengala sobre una cacerola con agua en caso de caerse de las manos no se quebra.
- Si la dentadura tiene mal olor, puede remojar 30 minutos en solución de una cucharada de blanquedor (Clorox) y una taza de agua. Enjuague bien la dentadura antes de poner en la boca.
- Debe sacar de la boca su dentadura 8 horas a lo menos todo los dias. Mientras la dentadura esté afuera de la boca, pongala en agua o enjuague bucal diluido.
- **No debe** de ajustar o limar la dentadura - puede ruinar la dentadura. **No debe** usar forros o adhesivos de dentaduras.

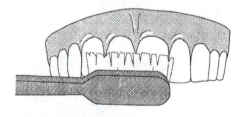
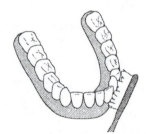

Visite el Dentista Para Lo Siguiente:
- Las citas regulares de ajuste
- Cuando tenga una ampoya en la boca que dura más de una semana
- Cuando se aflojen las dentaduras
- Una vez por año para revisar la salud de la boca y ajuste de la dentadura postiza.

Si necesita esta publicación en diferente formato, llame al numero
1-800-367-8939 (State TDD/TTY Relay) or 602-542-1866.

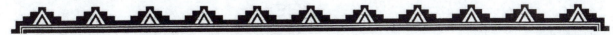

Oral Health
Fact Sheet

Dental Sealants

WHAT ARE DENTAL SEALANTS?

Dental sealants are thin plastic coatings which are applied to the chewing surfaces of the back teeth to prevent decay. Most tooth decay in children and teenagers occurs on the chewing surfaces with pits and grooves which tend to trap food and bacteria. Sealants fill in these pits and grooves so that bacteria cannot multiply and cause decay.

HOW ARE SEALANTS APPLIED?

Applying sealants is quite simple and may be done by a dental hygienist or dentist. First, the teeth are cleaned. Then the teeth to be sealed are dabbed with a very mild acid solution similar in strength to vinegar or lemon juice. This roughens the tooth surface slightly so that the sealant will bond to it. After the tooth is prepared, the sealant is painted onto the tooth. It flows into the pits and grooves and hardens in about 60 seconds. After sealing, bacteria cannot reach the pits and grooves and cause decay. Applying sealants requires no drilling or removal of the tooth surface.

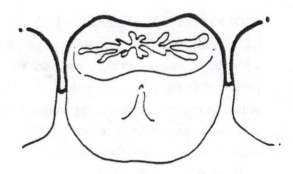

WILL SEALANTS MAKE TEETH FEEL DIFFERENT?

Sealants will not result in any change in bite because they are very thin and only fill the pits and grooves. At first they may feel bulkier, but a few days of normal chewing will wear the sealants into place.

HOW LONG WILL DENTAL SEALANTS LAST?

A sealant application can last as long as 5 years and often longer. Sealants should be checked regularly and reapplied if they wear off. Because teeth are more likely to decay when they first appear in the mouth, dental sealants are recommended for children and teenagers.

WHY IS SEALING A TOOTH BETTER THAN WAITING FOR DECAY AND FILLING A CAVITY?

Sealants help to keep teeth healthy by protecting them from decay. Decay destroys parts of the tooth. Each time a tooth is filled or a filling is replaced, more tooth is lost. Silver fillings last about 6 - 8 years before they need to be replaced. Using sealants saves time and money and helps to keep teeth healthy.

If you need this publication in alternate format, please contact us with your needs at
1-800-367-8939 (State TDD/TYY Relay) or 602-542-1866

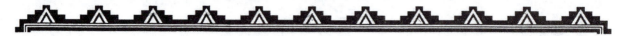

Oral Health
Fact Sheet

Sellantes Dentales

¿QUÉ SON LOS SELLANTES DENTALES?

El sellante dental es una capa fina de plástico que cubre y protege las superficies de las muelas posteriores. El sellante cubre las agrietas y no permité que entre la bacteria y la comida. Los sellantes se recomiendan para niños y jovenes porque son las edades más beneficiadas antes de que las muelas seán afectadas por caries.

¿CÓMO SE APLICAN LOS SELLANTES?

La aplicación de sellantes es muy sencillo y puede ser llevado a cabo por un higienista o dentista. Primero el diente se limpia y se seca. El sellante se le pinta encima llenando las agrietas y endureciéndose solo en un minuto. Al aplicar sellantes no se requiere myecciones y no es doloroso.

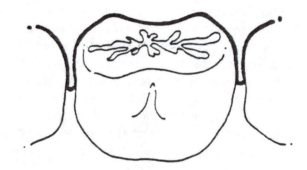

¿LOS SELLANTES HACEN LAS MUELAS SENTIR DIFERENTE?

No. Los sellantes son muy finos y no cambian la mordida. De vez en cuando las muelas se sienten mas altas pero esto se quita en dos o tres dias con solo masticar normalmente.

¿CUÁNTO TIEMPO DURAN LOS SELLANTES?

Una sola aplicación de sellantes dura cinco años o mas. Sellantes pueden ser revisados durante un examen dental general y ser cambiados cuando estén gastados.

¿PORQUÉ ES MEJOR LOS SELLANTES PARA PREVENIR QUE ESPERAR LAS CARIES O RELLENOS?

Poner sellantes en los dientes sanos hoy le ahorrará dinero y dolor mañana. Obtener los sellantes es la prevención de las caries dentales. Cuestan menos los sellantes que empastar o curar una carie.

Si necesita esta publicación en diferente formato, llame al numero
1-800-367-8939 (State TDD/TTY Relay) or 602-542-1866.

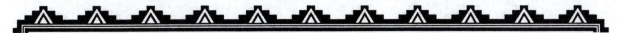

Oral Health Fact Sheet

Flossing Your Teeth

- Dental health begins with good oral hygiene. Proper toothbrushing helps to remove the germs that live on your teeth (called plaque), from the outside, inside and chewing surfaces of your teeth. But plaque will still remain on your teeth unless dental floss is also used.

- Flossing will remove plaque from **between** your teeth, especially in those hard-to-reach areas **under the gumline**. By combining the use of dental floss with toothbrushing to thoroughly remove plaque each day, you will be able to help prevent cavities and an infection in your gums called periodontal disease or gum disease.

How to Floss:

First wrap an 18-inch piece of floss around the middle finger of each hand.
Hold about an inch of floss tightly between your thumb and forefinger.

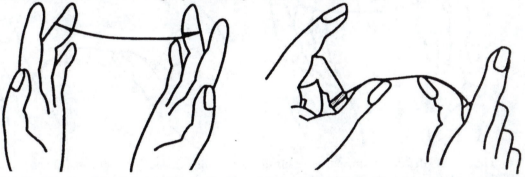

Gently slide the floss between the teeth. Be certain not to snap the floss in, or you may hurt your gums. Press the floss against one side of the tooth and move the floss up and down the tooth several times, being sure to reach under the gumline.

Floss both sides of every tooth. When you move on to the next tooth, be sure to use a clean section of the floss.

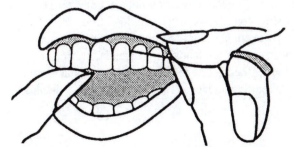

Your gums may bleed slightly the first few days you use dental floss. They will become healthier if you keep flossing. If it is hard for you to use floss, try a floss holder that you can buy at a drug store or pharmacy. It is recommended that you regularly visit a dental office to maintain the health of your teeth and gums.

If you need this publication in alternate format, please contact us with your needs at
1-800-367-8939 (State TDD/TYY Relay) or 602-542-1866.

Oral Health Fact Sheet

Usar Hilo Dental

• La salud dental comienza con buena higiene oral. El cepillar apropiadamente ayuda a eliminar la placa de las superfices externas, internas y de masticacíon de sus dientes, pero placa todavía queda en los dientes sin el uso del hilo dental.

• Usar el hilo dental quita la placa **entre** los dientes y **debajo de la encía**, adonde no llega el cepillo de dientes. La combinación del hilo y el cepillar todo los dias le ayuda prevenir las caries y infección en la encía nombrada periodontitis.

Cómo usar el hilo dental:

Enrolle 18" de hilo dental alrededor de sus dedos medios.
Dentenga una pulgada entre el dedo gordo y el dedo medio.

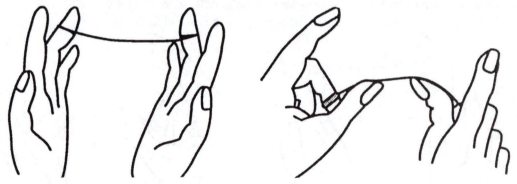

Guíe el hilo dental suavamente entre sus dientes. Tenga cuidado no lastimarse al entrar con el hilo. Mueva el hilo suavemente, hacia arriba y hacia abajo contra el diente y debajo de la encía.

Limpie los dos lados de cada diente. Use una parte nueva del hilo cada vez que cambie a otro diente.

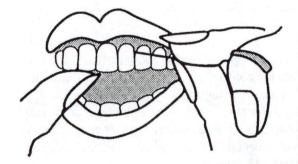

La encía le puede sangrar un poca al empezar por primeras con el hilo. Siga usando el hilo - en tiempo la encía sanará. Si tiene dificultades usando el hilo, compre un mango en la tienda o farmacia. Se le recomenda que visite regularmente una oficina dental para mantener la salud de su encías y dientes.

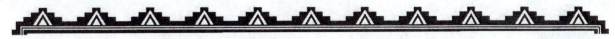

Oral Health Fact Sheet

Fluoride to Prevent Tooth Decay

What is Fluoride?

Fluoride is a mineral your body needs to grow and be healthy. Fluoride makes teeth and bones strong, and it protects your teeth against decay. It can be found naturally in all soil, plants, animals and water.

How Does Fluoride Help Your Teeth?

Fluoride is needed for infants and children - when teeth are still forming under the gums. The fluoride swallowed at this time, in water or from vitamins that contain fluoride, deposits itself into the outer part of the tooth and makes the tooth stronger and better able to fight decay.

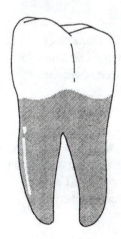

Fluoride also works <u>after</u> the teeth erupt, and are present in your mouth. At this time, fluoride from water, food, toothpaste, mouthrinses, and fluoride treatments received in a dental office, wash over the teeth and help to prevent decay or even stop small areas of decay that have already started. The fluoride minerals make the outer surface of the teeth stronger.

What is the Best Way to Get Fluoride?

Even though natural fluoride is found in food, plants, animals and water, the amount is usually too low to provide the best protection from decay. Many Arizona communities add a small amount of fluoride to their water supply so the best protection will be provided. This is called water fluoridation. Drinking fluoridated water from birth can reduce decay by 40 - 65%.

If a community does not have the benefits of water fluoridation, a dentist or physician can write a prescription for a vitamin with fluoride, in a tablet or drops. For best results, these tablets or drops should be taken from 6 months of age through 14 years of age.

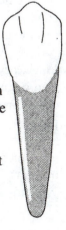

Many Arizona schools that do not have enough fluoride in their drinking water supply offer a fluoride mouthrinse program . The children that participate in this program swish with a fluoride mouthrinse once a week in their classroom. This program has been shown to reduce decay by 35%.

Another way to get fluoride is through dental products such as toothpastes or mouthrinses that have the seal of the American Dental Association on their label. These products are good for children and adults, whether or not they drink fluoridated water.

If you need this publication in alternate format, please contact us with your needs at
1-800-367-8939 (State TDD/TTY Relay) or 602-542-1866.

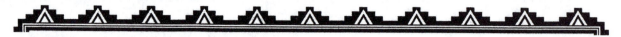

Oral Health
Fact Sheet

Fluoruro Para Prevenir Caries Dentales

¿Qué es Fluoruro?

Fluoruro es un mineral que el cuerpo necesita para crecer y fortalecer. El fluoruro hace los dientes y huesos fuerte, y protege contra caries. El fluoruro se encuentra naturalmente en todo tierra, plantas, animales, y el agua.

¿Cómo Ayuda Los Dientes El Fluoruro?

Fluoruro es necesario para los niños cuando los dientes se están formando bajo las encías. El fluoruro tragado durante este tiempo, sea en agua or vitaminas de fluoruro, se deposita alrededor del diente haciendolo más fuerte contra las caries.

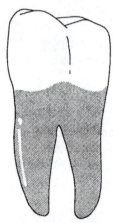

Fluoruro también trabaja después de salir los dientes en la boca. Durante este tiempo, fluoruro del agua, comida, pasta, enjuagues, or tratamientos de fluoruro en oficina dental, baña los dientes y ayuda prevenir caries y puede cesar caries pequeñas. Los minerales de fluoruro hacen fuerte el exterior del diente.

¿Cuál Es El Mejor Modo de Obtener Fluoruro?

Aunque hay fluoruro naturalmente en comida, plantas, animales, y en el agua, no es suficiente para proteger adecuadamente. Muchas ciudades en Arizona le ponen fluoruro en el sistema de agua para tener el major nivel de protección. Esto se nombra fluorización. Tomando agua con fluoruro desde nacimiento puede reducir caries de 40 - 65%.

Si la comunidad no tiene el beneficio de fluorización, un dentista o médico puede recetar vitaminas con fluoruro en gotas o tabletas. Para mejores resultados debe tomar las gotas o tabletas de seis meses hasta catorce años de edad.

Muchas escuelas en Arizona que no tienen suficiente fluoruro en el agua potable ofrecen un programa de fluoruro en enjuague. Los niños que participan en el programa enjuagan con fluoruro una vez por semana en la clase. Este programa aparace reducir caries por 35%.

Otras modo de obtener fluoruro es por medio de productos como pasta dental o enjuagues que llevan sello de American Dental Association. Estos productos son buenos para niños y adultos aunque si o no tomen agua con fluoruro.

Si necesita esta publicación en diferente formato, llame al numero
1-800-367-8939 (State TDD/TTY Relay) or 602-542-1866.

Oral Health Fact Sheet

Oral Cancer

Oral cancer will be found in an estimated 30,000 Americans this year, and will cause close to 8,000 deaths. Only half of those people with the disease will live more than five years.

Who Is At Risk for Developing Oral Cancer?

People who use tobacco and excessive alcohol increase their risk of oral cancer. People who spend a great deal of time in the sun may also have a higher risk for lip cancer.

More than 90% of all oral cancers are found in people over the age of 45, but oral cancer can happen at any age. Men develop oral cancer twice as often as women, and it occurs more often in African-Americans than in whites.

What Are the Symptoms of Oral Cancer?

If it is found and treated early, deaths from oral cancer can be reduced. Changes in your mouth that may be the start of oral cancer often can be seen and felt easily. A person can find these changes by doing a monthly exam of their mouth. Look for these signs, which are some of the warning signs of oral cancer:

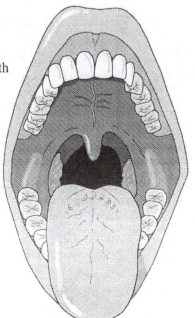

• A sore in your mouth that bleeds easily and does not heal

• A lump or thick spot in your cheek that can be felt with your tongue

• A white or red patch on your gums, tongue, or anywhere in your mouth

• Soreness or a feeling that something is caught in your throat

• Difficulty chewing or swallowing your food

• Difficulty moving your jaw or tongue

• Numbness of your tongue or other parts of your mouth

• Swelling of your upper or lower jaw that causes your dentures to fit poorly or hurt your mouth

These signs are not sure signs of cancer. They can also be caused by many other conditions. It is important to see a dentist or physician if any of these problems last more than 2 weeks. Pain is usually **NOT** a sign of oral cancer. Annual visits to a dental office are recommended for a professional oral cancer examination.

If you need this publication in alternate format, please contact us with your needs at
1-800-367-8939 (State TDD/TTY Relay) or 602-542-1866.

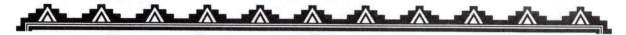

Oral Health Fact Sheet

Cáncer Oral

Encontrarán cáncer oral en estimado 30,000 Americanos éste año, y causará casi 8,000 muertes.

¿Quién Corre El Arriesgo De Contraer Cáncer Oral?

Los que usan el tabaco o alcohol en excesivo corren más arriesgo en contraer cáncer oral. Los que pasan mucho tiempo en el sol arriesgan cáncer en los labios.

Más de 90% de todos cánceres se encuentran en personas mayores de 45 años, pero el cáncer ocurre a cualquier edad. Ocurre dos veces más en los hombres que en las mujeres, y más en la gente negra que en la gente blanca.

¿Cuales Son Las Síntomas Del Cáncer Oral?

Encontrado y tratado temprano, las muertas de cáncer se pueden reducir. Cambios en la boca que pueden ser empiezos del cáncer se pueden ver y sentir muy facíl. La persona puede examinar la boca mensualmente. Busque estas síntomas que pueden indicar el cáncer oral:

- Una ampoya en la boca que sangra y no le sana

- Un bulto en el cacheta que puede sentir con la lengua

- Un parche blanco o rojo en las encías, lengua, o otro lugar en la boca

- Dolor de garganta o como que tiene algo en la garganta

- Dificultades en masticar o comer

- Dificultades en mover la lengua o quijada

- Sentir dormido la lengua o otras partes de la boca

- Hinchazón en la quijada que causa que no le quede bien la dentadura postiza

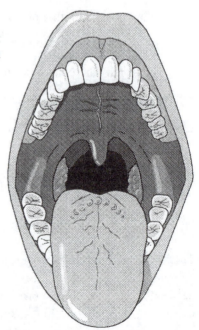

Estas síntomas no son seguras de que es cáncer. Pueden ser otra condición. Es muy importante ver un dentista o doctor si siguien más de dos semanas. Dolor casi **NUNCA** indica cáncer. Visitas anualmente a una oficina dental se le recomenda para el examen profesional de cáncer oral.

Si necesita esta publicación en diferente formato, llame al numero
1-800-367-8939 (State TDD/TTY Relay) or 602-542-1866.

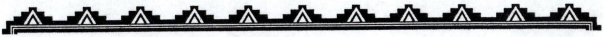

Oral Health Fact Sheet

Oral Injury Prevention-Mouthguards

- A mouthguard is a horseshoe-shaped, soft plastic device used to protect the teeth, lips, gums and cheeks from injuries which occur when playing many different sports.

- A recent survey of Arizona high-school interscholastic coaches revealed that mouth injuries (cut lips or broken teeth) are fairly common, and more than half of the athletes do not wear mouthguards.

- Mouthguards have been found to prevent more than 200,000 mouth injuries a year.

- Several studies suggest that mouthguards reduce the number of concussions by decreasing the force of injuries.

- There are three types of mouthguards:
  - Stock - ready to wear
  - Mouth formed - boil first and then bite to fit
  - Custom made - made by a dental professional from an impression made of your teeth

- Mouthguards can range in price from $1.00 to $100.00, and the money they can save you from repairing injuries to your mouth is well worth the investment.

- After using a mouthguard, it should be rinsed with water and stored in a rigid container with holes in it to allow the mouthguard to dry. Mouthguards can last for more than one season when cared for properly.

- The American Dental Association and other sports dentistry groups recommend the use of mouthguards in all organized team sports where a mouth injury can occur. This includes football, soccer, baseball, softball, basketball, volleyball and wrestling.

If you need this publication in alternate format, please contact us with your needs at
1-800-367-8939 (State TDD/TTY Relay) or 602-542-1866.

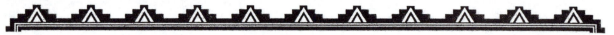

Oral Health Fact Sheet

Prevención de Perjuicio Oral-Guardabocas

- El guardaboca es un aparato de plástico suave que protegé los dientes, labios, encías y cachetes de daño que puede ocurrir jugando varios deportes.

- Una reciente encuesta de entrenadores de escuelas secundarias en Arizona revela que perjuicios orales (labios o dientes rotos) son muy común, y que más de la mitad de atletas no usan los guardabocas.

- Los guardabocas han prevenido más de 200,000 perjuicios orales al año.

- Varios estudios sugieren que guardabocas reducen la cantidad de concusiónes con reducir la fuerza del perjuicio.

- Hay tres tipos de guardabocas:
    De Surtido - listo para usar
    Formado Con La Boca - debe hervir luego morder
        para ajustar
    Echo Especialmente - echo por un dentista de
        impresiónes de sus dientes

- Los guardabocas pueden costar de $1.00 hasta $100.00. El dinero que se ahorra en tratar los daños a la boca lo hace una buena inversión.

- Después de usar el guardaboca, debe enjuagarlo con agua y ponerlo en un contenedor rígido con hoyos para poder secarlo. Los guardabocas pueden durar más de una estación con cuidado adecuado.

- La Asociación Dental Americana y otros grupos dentales recomiendan el uso de guardabocas en todo deportes donde puede ocurrir perjuicio a la boca. Incluye fútbol, soccer, béisbol, basketbol, balonvolea, y lucha.

Si necesita esta publicación en diferente formato, llame al numero
1-800-367-8939 (State TDD/TTY Relay) or 602-542-1866.

Oral Health Fact Sheet

Quitting Spit Tobacco

Before You Quit:
• Change to a brand you don't like
• Postpone your first chew of the day by 1 hour for a few days, then by 2 hours, then by 3 hours, etc.
• Set a date for quitting

When You Quit:
• Get rid of all your tobacco
• Tell everyone you know that you are quitting
• Have sugarless gum available for when you have the urge to chew
• Save the money you would have spent on tobacco and treat yourself to something you wouldn't usually purchase

When You Have the Urge to Use Tobacco, Do One of These Activities Instead:
• Take a walk or exercise with a friend
• Drink a glass of water

If You Feel You Need More Assistance With Quitting:
• Talk to your dental professional or physician
• Call the American Cancer Society at 1-800-227-2345
• Call the Arizona Lung Association at (602) 458-7505

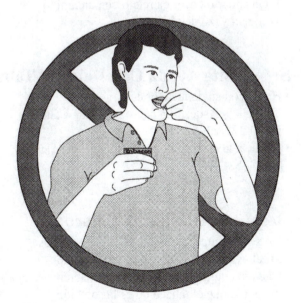

After You Quit:
• Don't worry if you are more sleepy or irritable than usual; these symptoms should go away.
• When you're in a tense situation, try to keep busy. Tell yourself that chewing won't solve the problem.
• Don't give up. **YOU ARE WORTH IT!**

If you need this publication in alternate format, please contact us with your needs at
1-800-367-8939 (State TDD/TTY Relay) or 602-542-1866.

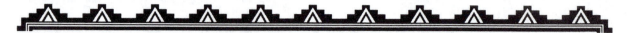

Oral Health Fact Sheet

Dejar El Uso De Tabaco Mascado

Antes De Parar:
- Cambie a una marca que no le guste
- Posponga el primer mascado del dia una hora por unos cuantos dias, después por dos horas, luego tres horas, etcétera
- Fije cita para dejar de usar tabaco mascado

Cuando Ya Lo Deje:
- Debe tirar todo el tabaco
- Deje saber a todos que dejo el tabaco
- Mantenga chicle sin azúcar para cuando le de ganas de mascar tabaco
- Compre algo para ud. mismo con el dinero que se horró en no comprar el tabaco

Cuando Le De Ganas De Mascar El Tabaco, Haga Otra Cosa:
- Vaya andar o hacer ejercicio con un amigo
- Tome un vazo de agua

Si Necesita Ayuda Con Dejar El Tabaco:
- Hable con su dentista or doctor
- Llame a la Asocación de Sociedad de Cáncer:
  1-800-227-2345
- Llame a la Asocación de Pulmónes de Arizona:
  (602) 458-7505

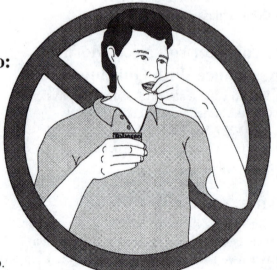

Después De Dejar El Tabaco:
- No se preocupe si tiene más sueño o es más irritable que antes, se le quitará en tiempo.
- Cuando tenga momentos tensos, mantengase ocupado. Recuerde que el tabaco no es la solución.
- No se de por vencido. **¡UD. LO VALE!**

Si necesita esta publicación en diferente formato, llame al numero
1-800-367-8939 (State TDD/TTY Relay) or 602-542-1866.

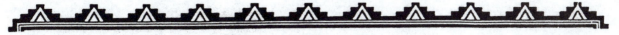

Oral Health Fact Sheet

Office of Oral Health

Arizona Department of Health Services
Community & Family Health Services
1740 W. Adams, Room 10
Phoenix, AZ 85007-2670
(602) 542-1866

Periodontal Disease

• Periodontal disease, also known as gum disease, is an infection that attacks the bone and gums that support your teeth. It is the most common cause of tooth loss in adults.

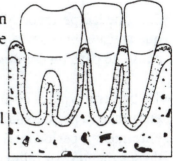

This is how gums and bone look in a healthy mouth.

• Bacteria in your mouth, called plaque, is the major cause of periodontal disease. Other things can contribute to periodontal disease such as the general condition of your teeth, your nutrition and general health, habits and emotional stress.

• If the bacteria is not removed regularly by brushing and flossing, it can harden into tartar, also called calculus. The rough surface of this calculus will help more bacteria to stay close to your teeth and under the gumline.

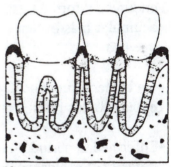

Notice how tartar, also known as calculus, has started to build up on these teeth. Bacteria live on its rough surface.

• This bacteria makes products that can harm your gums and the bone around your teeth.

• Periodontal disease is painless, and in the early stages it is difficult to detect. Common early warning signs of periodontal disease may include bad breath and tender or swollen gums that bleed when you brush and floss your teeth.

• Periodontal disease can be prevented with proper dental care from an early age, including brushing, flossing and regular dental visits for treatment from a dental hygienist and dentist. Caught in the early stages, periodontal disease is easy to treat.

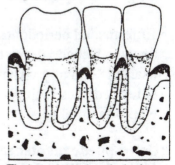

The bacteria on the calculus has caused these teeth to lose some of their bony support and has also caused the gums to shrink away from the teeth.

You can keep your teeth and mouth healthy for a lifetime! Ask your dental hygienist and dentist to evaluate the health of your gums.

If you need this publication in alternate format, please contact us with your needs at
1-800-367-8939 (State TDD/TTY Relay) or 602-542-1866.

Oral Health Fact Sheet

Enfermedad Periodontal

• Enfermedad periodontal o enfermedad en la encía es infección que ataca el hueso y la encía que soporta los dientes. Es la cause de pérdida del diente más común en adultos.

• La bacteria o placa en la boca es la mayor causa de enfermedad periodontal. Otras cosas pueden contribuir a la enfermedad periodontal - como sus alimentos, las condiciónes de sus dientes, su salud en general, y tensión emocional.

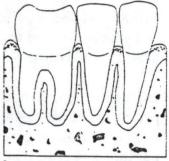

Las encías se ven así en la boca saludable.

• Si no quita la bacteria con cepillar y usar el hilo, se endurece y forma sarro o cálculo. El sarro áspero ayuda acumular más bacteria y placa junto al diente y debajo de la encía.

• La bacteria produce depósitos que le hacen daño a las encías y a los huesos que soportan los dientes.

• Enfermedad periodontal no es doloroso y a primeras es difícil detectar. Señales más común de la enfermedad periodontal incluyen el mal aliento y encías doloridas o encías que sangran al cepillar.

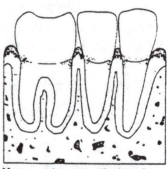

Nota que el sarro o cálculo se ha formado sobre el diente. La bacteria vive en lo áspero.

• Enfermedad periodontal se puede prevenir con cuidado dental adecuado desde temprano edad. Incluyen cepillar, usar hilo dental y visitas regulares con el dentista. La enfermedad es fácil para tratar si se alcanza en las etapas tempranas.

¡Usted puede mantener sus dientes y boca saludables por vida! Pregunte a su higienista or dentista por un examen de la salud de sus encías.

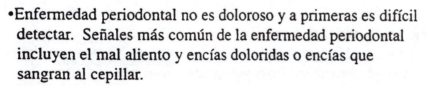
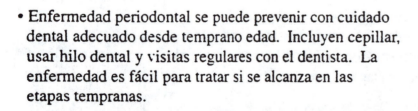
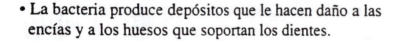
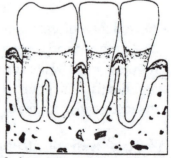

La bacteria ha causado que los dientes pierdan su soporto del hueso y las encías se encojen del diente.

Si necesita esta publicación en diferente formato, llame al numero
1-800-367-8939 (State TDD/TTY Relay) or 602-542-1866.

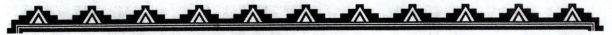

Oral Health
Fact Sheet

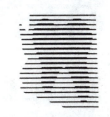

Tobacco Facts

- The nicotine found in cigarettes and in spit tobacco is a powerful, addictive drug that acts on several parts of the body. Once addicted, it becomes difficult, but not impossible, to quit using spit tobacco or to stop smoking.

- The use of tobacco products is not only addicting, but is directly related to a number of health problems and diseases. A few of the oral health problems smokers or spit tobacco users can develop are:

black hairy tongue	ground-down teeth	cancer of the palate
gum disease and loss of teeth	bad breath	cancer of the tongue
brown, stained teeth	receding gums	cancer of the lip
gum ulcers	cancer of the esophagus	cancer of the cheek

- Some of the harmful ingredients found in tobacco are:

- nicotine	- arsenic	- cyanide	- pesticides	- soot
- fertilizer	- dead bugs	- manure	- formaldehyde	- dirt

- At least 19 different types of cancer-causing substances, called nitrosamines, are found in tobacco products.

- Oral cancer is serious - when it spreads to the lymph nodes in the neck, it is often deadly.

- Spit tobacco is NOT a harmless alternative to smoking - it is just as hazardous to your health as cigarettes. Protect your health - avoid **all** tobacco products.

- The risk of developing lung cancer is ten times greater for smokers than non-smokers. Also, breathing second-hand smoke (someone else's smoke) can be as dangerous as smoking.

- Once you stop using tobacco products, within 20 minutes your blood pressure, pulse rate and skin temperature will return to normal. Within 8 hours, high levels of carbon monoxide in your blood will return to normal, and within a few weeks, your circulation will improve, your sense of taste and smell will improve, you will have fewer colds and more energy. **IT'S NEVER TOO LATE TO STOP!**

If you need this publication in alternate format, please contact us with your needs at
1-800-367-8939 (State TDD/TYY Relay) or 602-542-1866

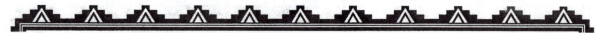

Oral Health Fact Sheet

Verdades del Tabaco

- La nicotina en el cigarro y en el tabaco de mascar es una droga poderosa y adictiva que actua en varios partes del cuerpo. El difícil pero no imposible de dejar usar el tabaco de mascar o fumar.

- El uso de tabaco no es sólo adictivo, pero también es relaciónado con varios problemas y enfermedades del cuerpo. Problemas que pueden contraer los que usan el tabaco son:

lengua negra pilosa	dientes gastados	cáncer en el paladar
enfermedad de las encías	peridida de dientes	cáncer en la lengua
dientes manchados	retracción de encías	cáncer de los labios
mal aliento	cáncer en el esófago	cáncer en los cachetes

- Varios ingredientes peligrosos en el tabaco son:

-nicotina	-arsénico	-cianuro	-fertilizante	-tierra
-pesticidas	-insectos muertos	-estercolar	-formaldehido	-tizne

- Nitratos también se encuentran en el tabaco. Hay 19 diferente tipos, y son la mayor causa de los diferentes canceres que ocurren.

- Todos los canceres son serios - ya que llege a los nodos linfas en el pescuezo puede ocurrir la muerte.

- El tabaco de mascar **NO ES** alternativa más sana que fumar - son igual en daño a la salud. Protega su salud - evite **TODO** producto de tabaco.

- El arriesgo de cáncer en los pulmones es diez veces más para los que fumar que para los que no fuman. También respirar el humo de los que fuman es peligroso como si también ud. fumara.

- Encuanto deje usar el tabaco, dentro 20 minutos la presión de sangre, pulso, y temperatura de piel se le volverá normal. Dentro 8 horas, el nivel alto de carbono monóxido en la sangra volvera normal. Dentro de unas semanas, la circulación mejorará, y el sentido de oler y sabor también mejorará. Ud. va tener menos catarros y más energía. **¡NO ES MUY TARDE PARA DEJAR EL TABACO!**

Si necesita esta publicación en diferente formato, llame al numero
1-800-367-8939 (State TDD/TTY Relay) or 602-542-1866.

Fresh Breath Assurance

-Kristy Menage Bernie, RDH, BS

– Bad breath affects everyone at one time or another and can be a source of embarrassment at any time. Simple techniques practiced on a daily basis will assure the freshest breath possible!

Bad Breath Culprits and Science

The term halitosis is commonly used when discussing bad breath and yet this term refers to odor produced by the stomach. In fact, 90% of bad breath is related to oral conditions and bacteria associated with gum disease. Bacteria collect on the back of the tongue and below the gum line where they produce odor-producing gases called volatile sulfur compounds (VSC). Unless these bacteria are removed and the VSC neutralized, odor will continue to be a problem.

Research has confirmed that the best way to address bad breath is through daily oral hygiene practices, which not only include tooth brushing and flossing, but cleaning the tongue as well. The American Dental Hygienists' Association has identified tongue cleaning as one of the most effective means for fresh breath. Additionally research on gum disease has proven that control of bacteria on the tongue will not only resolve bad breath but may also be an important factor in over all oral health.

The Toothbrush is for the Teeth!

Methods to assure fresh breath incorporate mechanical hygiene practices and products that will affect associated bacteria and neutralize foul-smelling VSC. Thorough and effective tooth brushing and flossing will assist in removing bacteria build-up around the gums; however, the toothbrush is for the teeth! Scientists have recently proven that cleaning the tongue with a plastic scraper is more effective and safer than a toothbrush. While the toothbrush will reduce VSC readings by 45%, a plastic scraper will reduce 75%! In addition, those using a tongue cleaner had improvement in taste within 2 weeks. This stands to reason, applying highly flavored, abrasive toothpaste to the tongue is bound to impact taste. Finally, the toothbrush simply moves bacteria around the shag carpet-like texture of the tongue and will not be effective in bacteria biofilm removal.

Neutralizing Odor

To enhance the effect of toothbrushing, flossing and tongue cleaning, mouthrinses, tongue sprays and toothpastes can be used that are designed to affect bad breath bacteria and neutralize odor-producing VSC. Chewing gum and mints can also assist in maintaining fresh breath, however, they should be sugar-free. The best products for fresh breath include a full product line and give the opportunity to maintain fresh breath in a variety of ways.

Fresh Breath Assurance

As gum disease is a main bad breath culprit, routine professional dental hygiene care will assure you the freshest breath possible and a healthy smile. Your dental hygienist is uniquely qualified to address bad breath concerns and treat the causes as well as make product recommendation. In addition, the registered dental hygienist is the preventive and therapeutic specialist who will guide you on maximizing optimal oral health and ultimately total health!

Fresh Breath Tips

- Seek regular and professional dental hygiene care
- Sip water frequently throughout the day
- Use powered toothbrushes and flossers for maximum plaque removal
- Practice daily, gentle tongue cleaning after brushing and flossing
- Avoid sugar-containing chewing gum or mints
- Replace old fillings that may be trapping food and bacteria
- Use mouthrinses and tongue sprays that contain ingredients to affect bacteria and neutralize VSC
- Discuss fresh breath options with your dental hygienist
- It's as simple as: BRUSH – FLOSS – SCRAPE – RINSE – REFRESH!

Active Agents for Fresh Breath

- Zinc—the most recognized and effective VSC neutralizing agent
- Essential oils—proven antimicrobial agent affecting VSC producing organisms
- Chlorhexidine gluconate—broad-spectrum antimicrobial agent that also neutralizes VSC.
- Chlorine dioxide—proven VSC neutralizing agent
- Cetylpyridinium chloride—proven mild antimicrobial agent affecting VSC producing organisms
- Triclosan—proven mild antimicrobial agent affecting VSC producing organisms
- Combination of above agents to achieve antimicrobial and VSC neutralizing results

Putting Your Best Smile Forward: Tooth Whitening Options

- Kristy Menage Bernie, RDH, BS

- From tooth whitening to aesthetic dental veneers and crowns, smile enhancement represents a dramatic and effective way to improve ones appearance. The goal of whitening smiles is an age-old endeavor that today can be accomplished quickly, effectively and safely. While tooth whitening represents the quickest and most cost effective way to impact a smile the overabundance of whitening choices are not only confusing to mere mortals, but dental professionals as well!

Basic tooth whitening science begins with two types of whitening processes: peroxide based whitening and non-peroxide based stain removal. Peroxide based whitening products remove stain deep within the tooth structure as well as surface staining through an oxidation reaction from the peroxide. This procedure is best initiated and supervised by a dental professional since there are many different dental conditions that may or may not respond to whitening and include two treatment options: professionally supervised and/or administered. Professionally supervised options include overnight or day time wearing of a custom fitted tray in which the peroxide based agent is placed, while professionally administered includes chairside or in-office whitening for immediate results. Either process will assure the best and quickest possible outcome and smiles can be whitened up to 8 shades or more under the expertise of a dental professional in as little as one hour!

While there are peroxide based products available to the public via television or drug store, they are not always reliable due to a many variables such as acidic and runny solutions which are easily swallowed and cause damage to the teeth and boil and bite mouth trays which will not fit well or provide whitening solutions to the teeth. In addition, many over-the-counter options have not undergone the testing seen with professionally recommended products. Recently the American Dental Association issued a statement that over-the-counter peroxide based whitening products would not be eligible for consideration for the ADA Seal of Acceptance. The ADA'S Statement on the Safety and Effectiveness of Tooth Whitening Products states *"Only those products dispensed through the dental office are considered for the Seal because professional consultation is important to the procedure's safety and effectiveness"*.

While peroxide containing over-the-counter products are not considered for the ADA Seal program, non-peroxide based products such as toothpaste are eligible for consideration. These products work by removing superficial surface stain and are useful in maintaining professional whitening results. Additional products that may claim whitening benefits include toothbrushes, which work by physically removing stain, chewing gum, which may remove stain via chewing action, and even dental floss, which is impregnated with a mild abrasive to again, physically remove stain from between the teeth. Regardless of these options the shade improvement is far less dramatic then those seen with peroxide based solutions and significantly less then the results achieved through professionally supervised or administered options.

Whitening Options · Consumer Information

Product Type	How does it whiten?	How well does it work?	Cost	Other!
Professionally supervised and in-office procedures – Laser – Non-laser – Non-light-activated	Combination peroxide agents with either laser or "light" source activation. Immediate results within 1–2 hours.	Highly effective on a range of staining. Shade improvement of 6–10 shades with life-long results.	$450.00–$850.00	Some in-office procedures may require more than one appointment. Typical treatment involves whitening all teeth at one time, in one visit.
	High concentration of peroxide in trays or directly applied to the teeth for a period of time with results in 1–2 hours.	1–4 shade improvement seen. Both options may cause temporary sensitivity.	$50.00–$200.00	Useful to initiate whitening and may be used in combination with taker-home products.
Professionally supervised and dispensed: – Take-home products	Rapidly working professional concentration of peroxide based gels. Day-time or night-time wear.	Effective on many types of staining, including internal tooth discoloration. Shade improvement up to 7 shades with long-term results.	$250.00–$350.00	Customized whitening trays to fit individual mouth and tooth size. Thick gels that stay in place within the tray and contain agents to minimize tooth sensitivity.
Direct response/ TV / Internet: – Differing systems	Ranging concentrations of peroxide and viscosities.	Effectiveness varies depending on product. Many contain acid based agents which may damage the teeth.	$30.00–$100.00	Lack of customized trays may lead to swallowing of whitening product; unknown ingredients and unproven results.
Over the Counter Limited use products – Whitening trays – Whitening strips – Paint-on products	Low concentration peroxide-based product. Daytime wear in general, with new paint-on products for overnight use.	Can be effective on age-related staining with reported shade improvement up to 4 shades for 6 months of results for the strips and paint-on products and unknown shade change for other options.	$15.00–$50.00	System is not specific to each individual's tooth or mouth size. Many tray systems contain thin gels and are acidic. Products are generally used without the removal of surface tooth stain, thereby producing limited whitening benefit or results.
Over the counter Daily use products: – Toothbrushes – Toothpaste – Dental floss – Mouth rinse – Chewing gum	Mechanical or physical removal of surface stain. Some toothpaste and chewing gum also claim to "coat" the teeth to prevent new staining.	Effective on surface stains only. Temporary results with claims of 1–2 shade improvement.	$.75–$5.00+	May be useful in maintaining professional tooth-whitening results.

222

With all of these options it is imperative that those seeking optimal tooth whitening results seek the advise of a dental professional for a thorough assessment, dental examination and appropriate recommendation based on those findings. Additionally, a visit with your registered dental hygienist prior to any tooth whitening procedure, will assure maximum results through the removal of surface tooth stain, plaque and tartar or calculus. The registered dental hygienist is uniquely qualified to advise you on tooth whitening options as well as options to maintain whitening results. In addition, the registered dental hygienist is the preventive and therapeutic specialist who will guide you on maximizing optimal oral health and ultimately total health!

Fluoride Products for Home Use

Fluoride Rinses, Non-prescription (OTC)

Alcohol Content (6–12%)

* Fluorigard Anti-cavity Fluoride Rinse (Colgate)	0.05% NaF
Act Icy Cool Mint, Spearmint (Johnson & Johnson)	0.05% NaF
*Rite-Aid Anticavity	0.05% NaF
*NaFrinse Neutral/Daily Mouthrinse	0.05% NaF
*NaFrinse Acidulated Oral Rinse (Medical Products)	0.05% APF
*Ortho Wash (Omnii)	0.044% APF
*Phos- Flur Anti-cavity Fluoride Rinse (Colgate)	0.044% APF
*ProDent$_x$ (ProDentec)	0.044% APF
Karigel (Young Dental)	0.05% APF

Alcohol Free

*Act for Kids (Grape, Bubblegum) (J & J)	0.05% NaF
*Act Mint, Cinnamon (J & J)	0.05% NaF
*Act Plus Freshening (J & J)	0.05% NaF

Directions: 1x/day – 1 minute

Don't eat or drink for 30 minutes

Fluoride Gels, Non-prescription (0.4% SnF$_2$)

*Gel-Tin	(Young Dental)
*Perfect Choice	(Biotrol International)
*Kids Choice	(Massco)
*Plak Smacker	(Plak Smacker)
*Just For Kids	(Omnii)
Oral B Stop	(Oral B)
*Gel Kam	(Colgate)
Kids Kare (Pro Dentec)	

Directions: 1-2x/day – Brush 1 minute; swish 1 minute

Don't eat or drink for 30 minutes

Fluoride Rinses, Prescription

NaFrinse weekly fluoride rinse (Medical Products Lab.)	0.2% NaF
PreviDent Dental Rinse (Colgate)	0.2% NaF
CaviRinse (Omnii)	0.2% NaF

Fluorinse (Oral B)	0.2% NaF
NeutraGard Plus (Pascal)	0.2% NaF
ProDent$_x$ (ProDentec)	0.2% NaF

Directions: 1x/day or 1x/week – 1 minute
Don't eat or drink for 30 minutes

Perio Rinses, Prescription (when diluted, 0.01% SnF$_2$)

Gel-Kam Oral Care Rinse (Colgate)	0.63% SnF$_2$
PeiroMed (Omni Oral Pharmaceuticals)	0.63% SnF$_2$
Perfect Choice Perio Rinse (Biotrol)	0.63% SnF$_2$
StanGard Perio Rinse (Pascal)	0.63% SnF$_2$
Perio Check (Pro Dentec)	0.63% SnF$_2$

Fluoride Drops, Prescription

*Karigel-N gel (Young Dental)	1.1% NaF
*Thera-Flur N drops (Colgate)	1.1% NaF
Thera-Flur drops (Colgate)	1.1% NaF

Fluoride Paste and Gels, Prescription

Perfect Choice Brush on gel (Biotrol)	1.1% NaF
Prevident 5000 Booster (Colgate)	1.1% NaF
Prevident 5000 Plus (Colgate)	1.1% NaF
Prevident Gel (Colgate)	1.1% NaF
Phos-Flur Gel (Colgate)	1.1% APF
Control R$_x$ (Omnii)	1.1% NaF
Cavarest Gel (Omnii)	1.1% NaF
Neutra Care (Oral B)	1.1% NaF
NeutraGard Home Care Gel (Pascal)	1.1% NaF
NeutraGard Advanced Gel (Pascal)	1.1% NaF
ProDent$_x$ (ProDentec) Brush Gel	1.1% NaF
ProDent$_x$ (ProDentec) Plus Dentifrice	1.1% NaF

* ADA Accepted
These products are not accepted by the American Dental Association (ADA).

Systemic Fluoride: Supplemental Fluoride Dosage Schedule (mg/day), 1994

Domestic Water Fluoride Concentration (ppm)			
Age	< 0.3 ppm	0.3–0.6 ppm	> 0.6 ppm
6 months–3 years	0.25 mg/day	0	0
3–6 years	0.5 mg/day	0.25 mg/day	0
6–16 years	1.0 mg/day	0.5 mg/day	0

ppm = parts per million.

Tooth Talk Dental Vocabulary

Table A–1 presents several common dental terms, accompanied by phrases that can be used when explaining these words to children or adult learners. This information can be given to the classroom teacher to incorporate as spelling words or given to the students to use when writing creative dental stories. Words and phrases can also be incorporated into year-end review lesson games and activities (such as matching word and description).

Table A–1   Tooth Talk Dental Vocabulary for Children and Adults

Tooth Talk	Children	Adults
Abscess	Bubble on the gums	Gum, boil, localized infection
Acid	Liquid that burns holes in teeth, tooth dissolver, eats holes in teeth	Liquid that burns holes
Air–water syringe	Wind–water gun, air gun, squirt gun	Spray used in the dental office to rinse off the tooth and gums
Amalgam/alloy	Silver star, silver filling	Silver filling
Aspirator	Little straw, vacuum cleaner	Used to remove water and debris from the mouth.
Blood	Red, hem, pink, RBCs	Blood
Bone loss	Bone disappears	Bone dissolves, is destroyed, is infected and loss of tooth support
Calculus	Tooth rocks, barnacles, coral	Calcified plaque, tartar, hard deposits, barnacles, or stones.
Cavity, caries	Hole in tooth, sick tooth, rotten, cave in tooth	Hole in tooth from decay
Curet/scaler	Little toothpick to clean your teeth, tooth cleaner, little spoon	Dental instrument to clean your teeth
Curettage		Removes the diseased or infected tissue inside the tooth and around the gum
Decay	Caused by the plaque + sugar = acid on healthy tooth = decay = cavities	
Dental floss	Like a piece of thread, string used to clean in between the teeth	Waxed, unwaxed, or tape, thin string used to remove plaque in between the teeth
Disclosing agent	Food coloring dye—shows if teeth are clean or dirty, red paint	Liquid or tablet, used for coloring the plaque, to make it visible
Explorer	Like a toothpick, tooth counter, tooth feeler	Dental instrument, used to check the teeth for cavities and calculus
Fluoride	Tooth hardener, shield, vitamins, added to toothpaste to make teeth strong	Substance that makes the tooth harder and stronger
Gingiva	Gums, skin around the tooth	
Gingivitis	Weak, soft, sick gums and unhealthy, puffy, red gums	A disease condition of the gums, infection, swelling

(continued)

Table A–1   Tooth Talk Dental Vocabulary for Children and Adults (continued)

Tooth Talk	Children	Adults
Hurt/pain	Bother, uncomfortable	
Head and neck exam		Checking to make sure glands and tissues are normal (healthy)
Plaque	Sticky, film of invisible bacteria, germs, sugar bugs that cause holes in your teeth	Film or colonies of invisible bacteria
Pocket		Infection on the inside of the gums, hole between the tooth and gums
Prophy angle	Electric toothbrush used in a dental office to clean the tooth	Used with a rubber cup in the dental office to polish the teeth after cleaning
Periodontitis		Infection of gums and bone, puss, bleeding, advanced gingivitis
Recession		Shrinkage of gums, gums pull away from tooth
Root planing		Smooth the root surface, clean the root surfaces
Slow speed	Air whistle, Mr. Bumpy	
Saliva Ejector	Mr. Slurpy, Mr. Thirsty	
Stainless steel crown	Silver hat, tooth hat	
Sulcus	Space around the tooth, between the tooth and gums	Cuff around tooth, little flap, space between the tooth and gums
Topical	Flavored jelly stick	
X-ray	Black and white picture of your teeth	Radiographs, dental films of your teeth
Xylocaine	Sleepy juice	Anesthesia

Courtesy of Diane Melrose, RDH, BS.

Dental Health Educational Resources

Table A–2 is a detailed listing of several different types of resources that may be useful to the dental health educator who is planning presentations for children in grades K–6. Since prices are subject to change, it is best if you contact each source to obtain their latest catalog.

The following list of contacts is a reference guide. Most of these sites have consumer friendly and professional education materials and catalogs of videos, etc., to use for your presentations.

Table A–2 Selected Dental Health Educational Resources

Item and Description	Source
Flipchart	
Baby Bottle Tooth Decay Prevention Pictures and script, for individual or group discussion	American Dental Association 211 E. Chicago Ave. Chicago, IL 60611-2678 (800)947–4746 Fax: (312)440–3542
Toothtalk (1975) Grades K–3, pictures and script, lesson activities	American Society of Dentistry for Children 211 E. Chicago Ave. Chicago, IL 60611 (800)947–4746
Videos	
Parents Helping Parents A 4-minute video that describes baby bottle tooth decay (available in other languages)	Public Health Foundation WIC Program 583 Monterey Pass Rd. Monterey Park, CA 91754 (818)570–4149
BBTD: A Professional Guide A 12-minute video on prevention for caregivers and health professionals	Dental Health Foundation 4340 Redwood Hwy., #319 San Rafael, CA 94903 (415)499–4648
American Dental Association (1995) *Baby Bottle Tooth Decay Prevention* *Brushing Magic with Dudley and Dee* *Dudley in Nutrition Land* *Dudley Visits the Dentist* *Dudley's Classroom Adventure* *Flash That Smile* *The Haunted Mouth* *It's Dental Flossophy, Charlie Brown* *Toothbrushing with Charlie Brown*	American Dental Association 211 E. Chicago Ave. Chicago, IL 60611-2678 (800)947–4746 Fax: (312)440–3542

(continued)

Table A–2   Selected Dental Health Educational Resources (continued)

Item and Description	Source
Brochures	
Protect Your Child's Teeth	Dental Health Foundation (listed above)
Nutrition Education Materials	Dairy Council of Wisconsin Westmont, IL
Advice for Parents	American Dental Association (listed above)
Baby Bottle Tooth Decay	
Basic Brushing	
Basic Flossing	
Benefits of Sealants	
Diet and Tooth Decay	
Happiness Is a Healthy Smile	
Smokeless Tobacco	
Stages of Tooth Development	
Your Child's Teeth	
Posters	
Toothbrushing chart	American Dental Association
Flossing chart	(listed above)
Baby bottle tooth decay	
Progress of tooth decay	
Smokeless tobacco	
Youth posters (variety)	
Slides	
Today's Dentistry	American Dental Association
Everything you need for a community presentation	(listed above)
Books	
Growing Up Cavity Free by Stephen J. Moss, DDS; "A parents guide to prevention"	Quintessence Publishing Co. 551 N. Kimberly Dr. Carol Stream, IL 60188-1881 (900)621–0387
The Bully Brothers Trick the Tooth Fairy by Mike Thaler 1993	Available in most bookstores or by special order
Brush Your Teeth Please, by Joshua Morris	
The Magic School Bus,	
Inside Your Mouth (activity book) and	
A Trip to the Water Works, by Linda Beech	
The Very Hungry Caterpillar, by Eric Carle	
Loose Tooth, by Steven Kroll	
Supplies	
Big tooth model	ADA (listed above)
Big toothbrush	also available at Block Drug Company 105 Academy Street Jersey City, NJ 07302 (800)365–6500
Anti-tobacco/smokeless tobacco brochures, posters, and books	American Cancer Society (800)4–CANCER
Bright Smiles/Bright Futures Grades 1 and 3 and preschool	Colgate One Colgate Way Canton, MA 02021 (800)334–7734

Table A–2 Selected Dental Health Educational Resources (continued)

Item and Description	Source
Tooth stickers, notepads, borders, posters, etc.	Carson-Dellrosa's P.O. Box 35665 Greensboro, NC 27425 (800)321–0943
Teacher supplies	Consult local phone book
Posters	CREST
Video (Sparkel)	Procter & Gamble
Brochures	Oral Health Products
Toothbrushes	Professional Sales
Toothpaste	P.O. Box 148013
Dental health month	Fairfield, CA 45014-9923
Activity books	(800)543–2577
Stickers	
Bookmarks	
Chairside aid	Colgate Oral Pharmaceuticals
Dental care kits	One Colgate Way
Brochures	Canton, MA 02021
Toothbrushes	(800)225–3156
Toothpaste	
Floss	Oral B Laboratories
Mouth rinse	One Lagoon Dr.
Fluoride	Redwood City, CA 94065
Toothbrushes	(800)446–7252
Toothpaste	Johnson & Johnson
Floss/fluoride	Dental Care Divison
Fluoride	New Brunswick, NJ 08903
Toothbrushes	(800)526–3967
Floss	Plak Smackers
ACT	4015 Indus Way
Toothbrushes/covers	Riverside, CA 92503
Fluoride	(800)558–6684
Toothbrushing timers	Fax: (909)734–4750
Disclosing tablets	E-Z Floss
Gloves/masks	P.O. Box 2292
Floss/Floss holder	Palm Springs, CA 92263
Kits	CA: (800)227–0208
Toothbrushes	Nationwide: (800)458–6872

Recommended Dental Titles

Several books with a dental health focus can be recommended for use in the elementary school classroom. New titles are constantly being released, and the dental health educator should make an effort to review these resources periodically.

Corporate	Contact
Colgate Oral Pharmaceuticals	www.colgate.com
Dentsply Professional	www.dentsply.com
Discus Dental	www.DiscusDental.com
Flossbrite	www.flossbrite.com
Laclede Inc	www.laclede.com
Oral B Laboratories	www.Oralb.com
Procter and Gamble	www.dentalcare.com
Sunstar Butler	www.commerce.jbutler.com
GlaxoSmisthKline	www.dental-professional.com

Association and Dental Hygiene Related	Contact
A to Z Teacher Stuff	www.atozteacherstuff.com
American Academy of General Dentistry	www.agd.org
American Academy of Pediatric Dentistry	www.aapd.org
American Academy of Periodontology	www.perio.org
American Association of Orthodontists	www.braces.org
American Association of Public Health Dentistry	wwww.saphd.org
American Association of Women Dentist	www.womendentists.org
(Dental fact sheet on women DDS)	www.aawd.org
American Cancer Society	www.cancer.org
American Dental Association	www.ada.org
American Dental Hygienist Association	www.adha.org
American Public Health Association	www.apha.org
Calgary Health Region: Dental and Oral Health Prevention	www.calgaryhealthregion.ca
California Dental Association	www.cda.org
California Dental Hygienist Association	www.cdha.org
Caries Diagnosis Risk Assessment & Management	www.aapd.org
Children's Alliance	www.childrensalliance.org/ kidsteeth.htm
Dental Health Foundation	www.dentalhealthfoundation.org

Association and Dental Hygiene Related	Contact
Health Forums; Library of topics: (Dental health, fluoride, etc.)	www.healthforums.com
Keep Kids Happy (dental health)	www.keepkidshappy.com
Kinder Hive	www.kinderhive.net
Lost Tooth Pillow/happy Teeth	www.Dltk-kids.com
Medline Search	www.ncbi.nlm.nih.gov/PubMed
Ms. Flossys Dental Hygiene News	www.ms-flossy.com
National Center for Fluoridation Policy and Research	http://fluoride.oralhelath.org
National Dairy Council (united Dairy Industry of Michigan)	www.nationaldairycouncil.org or www.udim.org
National Museum of Dentistry	www.dentalmuseum. umaryland.edu
Oral Health American's National Spit Tobacco Education Program	www.nstep.org
Preschool Education (dental health)	www.preschooleducation.com
San Diego County Office of Education Smiles	www.sdcoe.k12.ca.us
Sites for teachers	www.siteforteachers.com
Smile City	www.smilecity.ca
The Association of Professional Piercers	www.piercing.org
Tooth fairy letters	www.letterhut.com
University of Maryland Medical Center, Oral Health Guide	www.umm.edu/oralhealth.htm
Zoo animal teaching aid	www.teachingaid.com

Government	Contact
Center for Disease Control	www.cdc.org
Association of Maternal and Child Health Programs	www.mchoralhealth.org (bright futures) www.mchb.hrsa.gov
Food and Drug Administration	www.fda.gov
National Oral Health Information Clearing House, National Institute of Dental and Craniofacial Research	www.nidcr.nih.gov
U.S. Department of Health and Human Services and U.S. Department of Agriculture	www.healthierus.gov www.MyPyramid.gov
National Health Information Center	www.health.gov/hhic
Arizona Department of Health Services	www.azdhs.gov
Fluoridation guidelines	www.cdc.gov/mmwr/preview/ mmwrhtml/rr501al.htm
Washington State Department of health (H.E.R.E. Materials)	www.doh.wa.gov

Table A–3   Recommended Dental Titles

Title	Author	Price ($)	Publisher
A Tooth is Loose	Trumbauer	4.95	Children's Press
Alfred Goes to the Hospital	Schanzer	5.95	Barron's
All About Our Bodies Our Teeth	NL (author not listed)	4.50	Heian International
Anna's Special Present	Tsutsui	10.95	Penguin USA
Arthur's Loose Tooth	Hoban	3.50	HarperCollins
Arthur's Tooth (book and cassette)	Brown	7.95	Little, Brown
Arthur's Tooth (hardcover)	Brown	14.95	Little, Brown
Arthur's Tooth (paperback)	Brown	4.95	Little, Brown
Arthur Tricks the Tooth Fairy	Brown	3.99	Random House
B. Bears Go to the Dentist	Berenstain	2.95	Random House
B. Bears Go to the Doctor	Berenstain	2.25	Random House
B. Bears Go to the Doctor (puppet)	Berenstain	2.95	Random House
B. Bears Visit Dentist (book and cassette)	Berenstain	5.95	Random House
Bear in the Hospital	Bucknall	11.95	Penguin
Bear's Toothache	McPhail	5.95	Little, Brown
Betsy and the Chicken	Wolde	4.95	Random House
Betsy and the Doctor	Wolde	4.95	Random House
Big Bird Goes to the Doctor	SESST	2.95	Western
Brush Your Teeth Please	NL	9.95	Random House
BSLS 43 Karen's Toothache	Martin	2.95	Scholastic Book Service
Creatures Brush Their Teeth			
Dad Are You The Tooth Fairy	Alexander	16.95	Ochard
Dear Tooth Fairy	Durant	14.99	
Dilly Goes to the Dentist	Bradman	9.95	Viking Penguin
Doctor De Soto	Steig		Scholastic
Dragon Teeth and Parrot Beaks, Even	Grohmann	20.00	Quintessence Publishing
Franklin and the Tooth Fairy	Bourgeosis	4.99	Scholastic Paperbacks
Going to the Dentist	Borgardt	8.95	Simon & Schuster
Going to the Dentist	Civardi	3.95	EDC
Great Zopper Toothpaste Cyda	Boch	2.50	Bantam
Hospital Journal	Banks	7.95	Penguin USA
Hospital Story	Stein	8.95	Walker & Company
How Many Teeth?	Showers	4.95	HarperCollins
How the Tooth Fairy Got Her Job	Henry	3.95	Purple Turtle
I want My Tooth	Ross	4.95	Kane/Miller Book
Just Going to the Dentist	Mayer	2.25	Western
Little Rabbit's Loose Tooth	Bate	4.99	Random House
Loose Tooth	Schaefer	3.99	Harper Trophy
Loose Tooth (hardcover)	Kroll	13.95	Holiday House
Loose Tooth (paperback)	Kroll	2.50	Scholastic Book Service
Maggie and the Emergency Room	NL	2.25	Random House
Martin and the Tooth Fairy 3	Chardiet-Maccarone	2.50	Scholastic Book Service
Missing Tooth	Cole	3.50	Random House
Mr. Rogers Going to the Dentist	Rodgers	5.95	Putnam's

Table A–3   Recommended Dental Titles (continued)

Title	Author	Price ($)	Publisher
My Dentist	Rockwell	3.95	Wm. Morrow
My Tooth Is Loose	Silverman	3.50	Penguin USA
Nice Try Tooth Fairy	Olsen		Aladdin
Open Wider:Ttooth School Inside	Keller	16.95	Henry Holt and CO.
Ready Freddy Tooth Trouble	Klein	3.99	Blue Sky Press
Rita Goes to the Hospital	NL	2.25	Random House
Rosie's Baby Tooth	MacDonald	12.95	MacMillan/Atheneum
Ruth's Loose Tooth	NL	5.95	Price, Stern, Sloan
Saber Toothed Cat	NL	5.95	Simon & Schuster
Serpent's Tooth	Paxson	4.99	Avon Books
Serpent's Tooth Mystery	Dixon	3.50	Simon & Schuster
Teeth	NL	3.95	Steck-Vaughn/ Raintree
Throw your tooth on the roof	Beeler	5.95	Houghton Miffin
Tooth Book	Lesieg	6.95	Random House
Tooth Fairy	Wood	3.95	Child's Play International
Tooth Fairy Book	Kovacs	9.95	Running Press
Tooth Gnasher Superflash	Pinkwater	3.95	Macmillan/Atheneum
Tooth Witch (hardcover)	Karlin	11.95	Harper & Row
Tooth Witch (paperback)	Karlin	4.95	HarperCollins
Toothpaste Millionaire	Merrill	4.95	Houghton Mifflin
Trip to the Dentist	Linn	9.95	HarperCollins
When I See My Dentist	Kuklin	13.95	Macmillan
Who Put That Hair In My Toothbrush?	Spinelli	3.50	Dell
Why Am I Going to the Hospital?	Ciliotta	12.00	Carol

NL = author not listed

Classroom Education Resources

Classroom dental health programs are an integral component of the development of the whole child. Dental health education programs that are part of the total health curriculum can have a positive impact towards reducing dental disease, the most widespread public health problem among California's school age population.

Pre-school

5 Simple Tips to Keep Children's Teeth Healthy and Strong
Fact sheet for parents from the California Dental Hygienists' Association

"Brush Up on Healthy Teeth"
Simple Steps for Kids Smiles. A tip sheet for parents, quiz and poster to color. Also available in Spanish.
www.cdc.gov/OralHealth/factsheets/brushup.htm

"Denta-Claus? Santa Floss? The Tooth Fairy?: Dental Books for Children"
An extensive guide to the books written for children about dental health.
www.lib.umich.edu/dentlib/about/exhibits/kids

"Let's Talk Teeth"
A teacher's resource for dental health education lesson plans and craft projects for preschool through kindergarten.
www.AtoZTeacherStuff.com/Themes/teeth/index.shtml

Primary Grades

Tooth Facts for Kids
Dental health information for children from the American Dental Hygienists' Association. Includes tooth facts for kids and interactive dental health games.
www.adha.org/kidstuff/index.html

Smile City
Dental health information for children from the Canadian Dental Hygienist's Association. Includes a special parent and teacher page, games and activities in French and English.
www.smilecity.ca/

Open Wide and Trek Inside
An oral health curriculum developed by the National Institutes of Health and the National Institute for Dental and Craniofacial Research designed for grades 1-2
http://science-education.nih.gov/customers.nsf/
ESDental?openForm&CS_21=false&

Dental Health Education Units for Kindergarten through First Grade
Includes book and video lists, songs, poems, language, math and art activites.
www.kinderhive.net/teeth.html

Dental Health Education Lesson Plans for Grades 1 through 5
A collection of lesson plans for dental health units from teacher and commercial resources.
www.AtoZTeacherStuff.com/Themes/teeth/index.shtml

The Truth About Teeth
Dental and general health information written for children from the Nemours Foundation Center for Children's Health. Topics include: tooth anatomy, oral hygiene, cavities, braces and bruxism.
http://www.kidshealth.org/kid/body/teeth_noSW.html

Snack Smart
An easy to read booklet on health snacking. Describes the decay process and includes a poster with tips for health snacking.
http://www.nidcr.nih.gov/NR/rdonlyres/EB5532D3-D259-40E1-ACFE-522DA23C2AB6/5016/SnackSmartforHealthyTeeth1.pdf

Milk Matters
A coloring book for young children focusing on the importance of calcium for healthy teeth.
http://www.nichd.nih.gov/milk/book0115/coloringbook0115.pdf

Middle and High School

Adolescent Oral Health
Fact sheet from the American Dental Hygienists's Association

National Institute of Health Office of Science Education
Curriculum supplements for middle and high school students
http://Science-education.nih.gov/

Taking Care of Your Teeth
Information directed towards adolescents from the Nemours Foundation. Includes general health subjects as well as dental health topics including oral hygiene, decay, diet, and bad breath.
http://kidshealth.org/teen/your_body/take_care/teeth.html

Tobacco Cessation Materials for the Classroom

Spitting into the Wind
The Facts about Dip and Chew
A brochure highlighting the health risks associated with spit tobacco use and addiction with advice for quitting
http://www.nidcr.nih.gov/HealthInformation/DiseasesAndConditions/SpitTobacco/SpittingIntoTheWind.htm

Spit Tobacco: A Guide for Quitting
A booklet written for young men who have decided to quit using spit tobacco. The pamphlet contains a quit plan as well as information on over the counter and prescription medications to help quit the nicotine habit.
www.nidr.nih.gov/health/newsandhealth/spittobacco

Take a Close Look at What the Tobacco Industry Won't Show You
A poster showing the effects of oral cancer.

http://www.nidcr.nih.gov/HealthInformation/DiseasesAndConditions/
SpitTobacco/TobaccoIndustryWontShowYou.htm

Campaign for Tobacco Free Kids
www.tobaccofreekids.org

Tobacco Education Clearing House of California
www.tecc.org/public
Materials available include: Loose the Chew Cessation Packet, Want to Quit
Chewing? Brochure, Chewing Tobacco Trading Cards, Friends Don't Give
Friends Cance, Lose the Chew Poster

Quitting Chew. A PDF fact sheet from California Smokers Helpline
http://www.californiasmokershelpline.org/Information/pdf_files/
Quitting_Chew.pdf

Oral Health America's National Spit Tobacco Education Program
www.nstep.org

Teaching Aids for Classroom Education Program

Classroom education aids from the American Dental Hygienists' Association
www.adha.org/shopping/patient.htm

Interactive Tools and Illustrations
Interactive teaching aids and original illustrations from the University of
Pennsylvania Simple Steps to Better Dental Health Website
www.simplestepsdental.com/SS/ihtSS/r.WSIHW000/st.31843/t.31843/
pr.3.html

Zoo Animal Teaching Aids
Puppet animals with dental models and an oversized toothbrush. Links to dental
poems, plays and classroom activities.
www.teachingaid.com

Source: ©2005 The California Dental Hygienists' Association—www.cdha.org

Glossary

Abscess Infection (pus) in the tooth tissue usually caused by bacteria.

Abutment teeth Surrounding teeth that are on either side of the missing. Teeth maybe used to anchor a fixed bridge or appliance.

Acid A compound having a sour taste that has the ability to destroy enamel.

Alveolar bone The bone which the teeth are set in.

Amalgam A filling material made of alloy, silver, tin, and mercury used to fill the teeth when the decay has been removed.

Anklysis Tooth permanently attached to the surrounding bone.

Anterior teeth Term that refers to all the front teeth: centrals, laterals and cuspids of both the maxillary and mandibular arch.

Apthous ulcer Canker sore.

Arch (dental) The horseshoe-shaped alveolar bone in which the teeth are set; maxillary and mandibular arches.

Bacteria (germ) A large group of one-celled microorganisms, many of which are disease producing (decay, periodontal disease).

Bicuspid (premolar) Permanent tooth in the dentition that has two (bi) cusp tips located in back of each cuspid. There is a first and second bicuspid in each arch. These teeth are used to tear and grind food.

Bruxism The clinching or grinding of the teeth, sometimes during sleep, that causes a wearing away of the occlusal enamel surface.

Calculus (tarter) Hardened plaque that has mineralized and adheres to the crowns and roots of the tooth surfaces; must be removed by a dental professional.

Canine tooth See cuspid.

Caries (tooth decay) A localized bacterial disease process which destroys tooth structures and produces a cavity.

Cavity The decayed portion of a tooth usually appearing brown in color; will leave a large hole in the tooth if the decay is not removed.

Cementum A calcified tissue which forms the outer layer on the roots of the teeth.

Composite Plastic/resin filling material used to restore the tooth surface after the decay has been removed.

Crown The top portion of the tooth that is covered with enamel and is visible above the gum line (clinical crown).

Cuspid (canine) A sharp pointed tooth located between the first bicuspid and the lateral incisor; used for tearing food; sometimes called the eye tooth.

Decalcify To remove calcium salts from the bone or teeth by a biochemical action. Some foods if left on the teeth long enough will cause the tooth area to decalcify over time, leaving white spots where the enamel should have been.

Decay To become impaired or rotted, as in a cavity.

Deciduous teeth 20 primary teeth that are shed at a certain age; baby teeth.

Dental assistant A professional in the dental office who assists the dentist or dental hygienist; may or may not be licensed.

Dental hygienists A professionally educated, licensed person who provides preventive services; may work in a dental office, public health, specialized practice, etc.

Dental (personal) A professional person who assists in the dental office usually in the front (makes appointments, finances, greets the patients, etc.).

Dental Public Health Specialty area that prevents and controls dental diseases through organized community efforts.

Dentifrice A cleaning substance, toothpaste or toothpowder, for the teeth; made with or without fluoride.

Dentin The hard, dense, calcified tissue that forms the body of the tooth underneath the enamel and the cementum.

Dentist (DDS or DMD) A professionally educated person licensed to provide services that provide care of teeth; DDS: Doctor of Dental Surgery; DMD: Doctor of Dental Medicine.

Dentures A set of artificial teeth.

Diet Food and drink taken daily as substance by a person.

Enamel The smooth, hard outer layer of the tooth that covers the crown portion.

Endodontist Specialist that deals with the diagnosis, treatment, and diseases within the dental pulp; may perform root canal therapy.

Eruption The process of teeth breaking through the gums.

Extosis A bony outgrowth (tori/torus) inside the oral cavity.

Extraction Removing or pulling a tooth from the alveolar bone/socket.

Filling A material (gold, silver, plastic, etc.) inserted in a prepared cavity in a tooth to replace the missing tooth structure.

Fissure A groove in the occlusal surface of the tooth caused by the imperfect enamel formation.

Fistula An abnormal passage/canal leading from an infected area.

Floss Dental string/yarn used to clean in between the teeth.

Fluoridation The adjustment of the fluoride content in the public water supply to prevent and reduce tooth decay.

Fluoride A compound mineral of fluorine and other elements used to prevent tooth decay; may be used as a varnish; in toothpaste, mouth rinses, vitamins, etc.

Fluoride (systemic) Liquid or tablet that is swallowed to provide fluoride within the body systems (fluoride added to the water).

Fluoride (topical) Gel, foam, liquid, or rinse applied on the tooth surfaces by the dental professional, used to help prevent tooth decay.

Furcation Area directly under the tooth crown of two or more root surfaces.

Gingiva (gums) The tissue which covers tooth roots and the alveolar bone of the maxillary and mandibular teeth.

Gingivitis Inflammation involving the gums and gingival tissue.

Gumboil (abscess) Inflamed and painful part of the gum tissue caused by an abscessed or diseased tooth.

Halitosis (mal odor) A oral health condition where the individual has consistently bad breath or mal odor coming from the oral cavity.

Impacted tooth A tooth embedded in the alveolar bone in such a way that it is not able to erupt.

Implant Prosthetic appliance to replace a single or multiple tooth root that is anchored into the alveolar bone; a crown is placed over the appliance.

Incisal Top/biting surface of the anterior teeth.

Incisors Any one of the four front teeth maxillary or mandibular; centrals: the two front teeth in both maxillary and mandibular arches; laterals: teeth situated on either side of the central incisors in both the maxillary and mandibular arch.

Malocclusion An irregularity of tooth position and poor fitting together of the teeth when the mouth is closed.

Mandible (mandibular) The lower arch in the oral cavity.

Mastication The act of chewing.

Maxilla (maxillary) The upper arch in the oral cavity.

Maxillofacial surgeon Specialist that deals with the diagnosis and surgical and adjunctive treatment of dental disease, injuries, etc., in the oral cavity.

Molar The three teeth in the back of the arch, starting with the first molar located behind the second bicuspid; used for grinding the food.

Neck/collar of the tooth Portion of the tooth where the enamel ends on the crown and the cementum begins on the root surfaces.

Nerve The nerve fiber (blood vessels) found in the pulp, which supplies the tooth with feeling and sensitivity.

Occulsal Top/biting surface of the posterior teeth.

Oral hygiene Cleanliness or proper care of the oral cavity.

Orthodontic appliance A device (retainer, head gear, etc.) used by the orthodontist to guide or straighten teeth into the proper alignment for chewing.

Orthodontist A professionally educated licensed dentist who specializes in providing care that deals with the prevention and treatment of malocclusion.

Partial denture An appliance that replaces one or more but not all the missing teeth.

Pedodontist Dental specialist that deals with the healthcare, prevention, and treatment of children's teeth from infancy to adolescent.

Peridontium The tissue that surrounds, supports, and attaches the teeth, gingiva, periodontal ligament, cementum, and the alveolar bone.

Periodontal Ligament A thin layer of tissue that surrounds the root structure of the tooth; the tiny fibers hold the tooth in place.

Periodontist Specialist who deals with treatment and prevention of gum diseases and tooth loss.

Periodontitis Inflammation of the gingiva surrounding the tooth structure which, if not treated, could result in the loss of the tooth; may cause foul odor, bad breath, abscess, etc.

Permanent teeth 32 permanent teeth: incisors, vuspids, bicuspids, and molars.

Pit A small indentation in the crown surface of the tooth.

Plaque Sticky film of bacteria.

Posterior Teeth in the back of the oral cavity: biscuspids, molars.

Prophylaxis The professional cleaning by a licensed individual to aid in the prevention of dental disease.

Prosthodontist Dental specialist who deals with restoring teeth, crowns, dentures, postoral cancer reconstruction, jaw joint problems, snoring, and sleeping disorders.

Protrusion Projection of the upper front teeth often caused by thumb sucking.

Pulp The core area of the tooth in which all the blood vessels, nerves, and connective tissue lie.

Pulpectomy Complete removal of the pulp and the pupal in the root of the tooth.

Pulpotomy Partial removal of the pulp (usually coronal).

Quadrant Any one of four parts or quarters of the dentition.

Root The part of the tooth that is normally beneath the gums and anchors the tooth in place.

Root canal The passageway in the root through which blood vessels and nerves enter the pulp chamber.

Saliva The clear, alkaline secretion from the glands discharging into the mouth that aids in preventing tooth decay.

Scaler A dental instrument used to remove the plaque and calculus from the tooth surface.

Sealant Plastic coating put on occlusal surfaces to prevent decay.

Sodium fluoride A chemical combination of sodium and fluorine.

Space maintainer A fixed or removable appliance used to replace missing teeth and hold that space in place until the permanent tooth or device is in place.

Stannous fluoride A chemical combination of tin and fluorine.

Subluxation Partial or incomplete dislocation of the tooth, usually due to accident.

Succedaneous teeth Primary teeth that will be shed and replaced by the permanent teeth; incisors, cuspids and first and second primary molars.

Supernumerary tooth Extra tooth may be erupted or unerupted.

Suppuration Formation of pus.

Tartar Hardened plaque that forms and adheres to the crowns and roots of the teeth.

Temporomandibular joint The hinge of the jaw in front of each ear; the mandible attaches to this area.

Wisdom tooth The third or last molar in the oral cavity.

Xerostomia Dryness of the mouth, which may be cause from medication and can lead to tooth decay.

X-ray/radiograph Radiation produced to form an image on the dental film when taken in the oral cavity; picture of the teeth

Xylitol Natural sweetener found in plants. Used in gums and other products. Dentally safe and low in calories.

Bibliography

American Dental Association. (1980). *Learning about your oral health: A prevention-oriented school program* (Vols. 1–4). Chicago: Author.

American Society of Dentistry for Children. (1975). *Tooth talk. A teacher's guide flip chart K–3.* Chicago IL: Author.

Nathe, Christine, Dental Public Health, Bowen Contemporary Practice For The Dental Hygienist Pearson Prentice Hall, New Jersey, 2005.

P.L. (1994). Teaching oral health in the classroom. *Dental Teamwork*, January–February, 26–27.

Brown, W. (1995). *Facts on water fluoridation.* Sacramento, CA: California Department of Health Services.

Children's Dental Disease Prevention Program, S.B. 111, Health and Safety Code §§ 360–375.5 (1979). Article 4.5 Children's Dental Disease Prevention Program.

Dembo, Myron H. (1994). *Applying Educational Psychology,* 5th ed. Longman Publishing Group.

FDA guidelines on Nutrition.

Hunter, M.C. *The Teaching Process,*_____.

Hubert, Jeannie, Xylitol: Magic in the making accessed 08-30-06 www.cdha.org

The Family School Partnership Act, AB2590 (1995, State of California).

Merriam-Webster's collegiate dictionary (10th ed.). (1993). Springfield, MA: Merriam-Webster.

Moss, S.J. (1993). *Growing up cavity free.* Chicago: Quintessence Publishing.

Renner, G. (1985). *The instructor's survival kit.* PFR Training Associates Limited.

U.S. Department of Health and Human Services, Public Health Service. (1991). *Healthy people 2000. National health promotion and disease prevention objectives.* Washington, DC: Author.

Yee, H. (1982). *Mini activity packet for teachers. State dental disease prevention program.* Sacramento: State Dept of CA.

www.keepkidshealthy.com   2005-07-30
www.umm.edu/oral health.htlm.   2005-07-30
www.doh.wa.gov.   2005-07-30
www.healthforms.com   2005-07-30
www.caringforkids.cps.ca   2005-07-30
www.healtheirus.gov   2005-07-30
www.CDC.org   2005-07-30 Guidelines Seniors
www.azdhs.gov   2005-07-30
www.cdha.org   2006-08-30
www.adha.org   2006-08-30
www.cda.org   2006-08-30

Index